ENERGETICS:

An Introduction to the Therapeutic use of Electromagnetic Energy

by

R.L. Worthy

KornerStone Books
6947 Coal Creek Pkwy
Suite 206
Newcastle, WA 98059
Ksbooks@execs.com

Published by

KornerStone Books
6947 Coal Creek Pkwy
Suite 206
Newcastle, WA 98059
Ksbooks@execs.com

Design and Layout: KornerStone Books

Unless otherwise stated, all images courtesy of The Hall of Records - KornerStone Books ©

Printed in the United States of America

The First Edition

ISBN: 978-0-9727627-4-8

This effort is dedicated to everyone with the intellectual dexterity and moral integrity to be worthy of it!

FIRST THINGS FIRST:

I HAVE NO FORMAL TRAINING IN ALLOPATHIC MEDICINE. WHAT'S MORE, **THIS IS NOT A BOOK ABOUT TREATING ANY SPECIFIC DISEASE**; E.G., AIDS, BREAST CANCER, HERPES, MENINGITIS, HEPATITIS, PROSTATE CANCER, ETC. THAT SAID, I AM A WORLD TRAVELER AND AUTODIDACTIC RESEARCHER OF HISTORY, CULTURAL ANTHROPOLOGY, AND THE FIELD OF ENERGETICS. THIS WORK IS ABOUT A SAFE AND **SCIENTIFICALLY PROVEN** METHOD TO ELIMINATE THE MICROORGANISMS WHICH CAUSE THE AFORE MENTIONED! FINALLY, THE LAW OF THE LAND REQUIRES THAT THE INFORMATION IN THIS BOOK BE INTENDED FOR RESEARCH AND/OR THEORETICAL PURPOSES ONLY—**AND NOT BE SEEN AS MEDICAL ADVICE** . . .

RL Worthy

Preface:

I have undertaken this effort to bring you the facts about a safe, simple and scientifically verified way to use electromagnetic energy to assist the body in the elimination of viruses, bacteria and parasites! While I believe the practice to be ancient in origin, vestiges of its use by Western Europeans date back to the 18th century CE. However, the champion of the 21st century re-emergence of this science is the accomplished American physicist Dr. Robert C. Beck DSc. Despite having many appellations through the ages, I prefer the blanket term of *Energetics* to describe the therapeutic use of electromagnetic energy. It is my sincere hope that the information in this book will prove as useful to you as it has been for me . . .

CONTENTS

Dedication   v

First Things First   vii

Preface   ix

Table of Contents   xi

Perception Vs. Reality   1

Warning: *The Use of Allopathic Medicine may be hazardous to your Health*   26

The Medical Industrial Complex   36

Who Is This Bob Beck?   54

Bob Beck Lecture: *Take Back Your Power Researchers*   60

What Does This Mean—Theoretically?   101

Conversation with an Energy Practitioner   116

CONTENTS
{cont}

Life & Electromagnetic Energy   128

Electromagnetic Energy & Health in History   145

Sexual Health   168

My Testimony   177

Epilogue   183

Glossary   185

Photo Credits   203

Bibliography   207

Index   220

Discount Order Form   229

Perception Vs. Reality

Perception Vs. Reality

While the roots of Northwestern Europe's formal empirical medicine can be said to date back to Medieval times (about 500 years ago) the truth is that mankind was practicing methodical results-based medicine millenniums before the Middle Ages. Despite the xenophobia and racism that permeates a good deal of Western academia today, objective researchers have made some rather extraordinary disclosures about the medical capabilities of the world's first scientific physicians!

Indeed, far from the stereotypical view of a few curious souls tossing bones in the air—the doctors of ancient Egypt and Mesopotamia were highly skilled and effective healers. It should be noted that these practitioners were also pharmacologists; <u>and let me be clear, their methodology was empirical and masterful</u>! For example, thousands of years before the rise of Greek civilization, Egyptian physicians were not merely performing intricate surgeries successfully—they had developed a safe and effective lactic acid contraceptive for women![1]

Indulge me for just a moment while I try to illustrate the disconnect between modern medical perception and the historical reality. Many of you have no doubt heard of the English physician William Harvey. Living in the 17th century CE, Harvey is widely celebrated in the West as the first person to discover that the human heart pumped blood to various parts of the body.

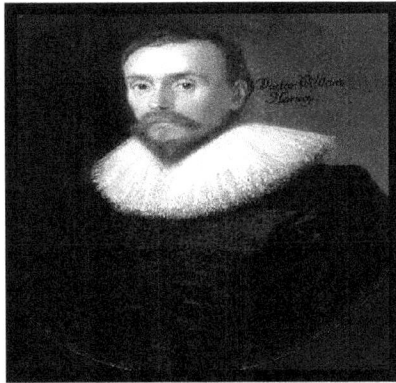

William Harvey c.1600 CE

---

[1] The Eber's Papyrus mentions the use of acacia, honey and dates to formulate a contraceptive for women. Today, chemists explain that these combined elements produce lactic acid—*a key ingredient in modern contraceptive gels!*

**<u>Before the life of Harvey (oft referred to as
"The Father of Cardiovascular Medicine")
Europe's medical community believed that
the human heart's principal function was to
heat the body through the conduction of
warm air</u>**.[2] While Harvey's discovery was laudable
and important, astute historians cannot help note
how late it was. You see, the ancient Egyptians were
well aware of the heart's role in blood circulation
and pulse 3500 years earlier!

Further, not only did they understand the
importance of the heart—they also wrote texts
which describe the anatomical purpose of many
organs! They saw the heart as the seat of human
physiology; and the blood stream was known as,
*"the conducting system of man in which all disease
originates."* Unlike the Western physicians of

---

[2] Osler, W., <u>The Evolution of Modern Medicine</u> & Bailey, R.,
<u>William Harvey – Father of Cardiovascular Medicine</u> (net)
These doctors thought blood was pumped by the lungs.

Harvey's age, they also considered blood to possess special or *magical* properties. A common Egyptian greeting was *"May your 'mtw' [vascular system] flourish!"* Remarkably, ancient writings dating to the 3rd century BCE—diagram and distinguish between human arteries, veins, glands and nerves![3]

Again, what's so profound about this (*on the Perception verses Reality tip*) is the heralded Greek physician Hippocrates (commonly celebrated today as *"The Father of Medicine"*) actually believed the liver to be the center of the human vascular system. That notwithstanding, medical historians explain:

[3] Budge, E.A., The Dwellers on the Nile pp. 196 - 198 & Stetter, C., The Secret Medicine of the Pharaohs pp. 28 – 32 & Heart, Encyclopedia of Religion Vol. VI, p. 234 & Dampier-Whetham, W., A History Of Science: And its relations with Philosophy & Religion p. 7 & Donnelly, I., & Sykes, E., Atlantis: The Antediluvian World p. 109 & Wilson, J., Culture of Ancient Egypt p. 56 & (Audio), Ancient African Medical Practices C. Finch 1992 & McGrew, R., Encyclopedia of Medical History p. 131 & Fagg, C., Ancient Greece p. 41 & Bowden, D., Who was Who in the Greek World p. 121 & Saunders, J., The Transitions From Ancient Egyptian to Greek Medicine p. 27, 30 & De Lubicz, R., The Temple in Man pp. 45 – 46, 106 - 107

"In medicine and surgery, the Egyptians recognized the importance of the heart and its relation to other parts of the body. They related the speed of a person's heartbeat to his general physical condition . . ."[4]

The fact that the Egyptians were mummifying their royalty 5,000 years ago clearly facilitated their unrivaled comprehension of human anatomy. For instance, the <u>Smith Papyrus</u> proves they were the first people to empirically study the human brain. From the documentation that presently exists, one can ascribe the absolute identification of all the

---

[4] Dampier-Whetham, W., <u>A History Of Science: And its relations with Philosophy & Religion</u> p. 7 & Egypt, <u>The World Book Encyclopedia</u> Vol. V, p. 2228g & Thornwald, J., <u>Science and Secrets of Early Medicine</u> p. 54 & Sedgewick, W., Tyler, H., & Bigelow, R., <u>A Short History of Science</u> pp. 31 – 32 & De Lubicz, R., <u>Sacred Science: The King of Pharaonic Theocracy</u> p. 98 & McGrew, R., <u>Encyclopedia of Medical History</u> pp. 47 - 48, 321 & Hobson, C., <u>The World of the Pharaohs</u> p. 128 & Maspero, G., <u>History of Egypt</u> Vol. VI, p. 70 & Ghalioungui, P., <u>Magic and Medical Science in Ancient Egypt</u> pp. 68 – 71 & Oates, J., <u>Babylon</u> pp. 180 - 183 & Smith, W., <u>Dictionary of Greek and Roman Biography and Mythology</u> Vol. II, p. 1009

regions of brain to the Egyptians. It is also safe to conclude that they would undoubtedly have begun to make basic observations about brain functionality millenniums before the emergence of the Greeks and Romans. According to De Lubicz, the Temple of Amen-Ra was designed and constructed so as to memorialize their anatomical comprehension!

Additionally here, a museum in Egypt possesses the cranium of an ancient Egyptian man who appears to have undergone successful brain surgery c. 2500 BCE. <u>I say successful because modern examination of the cranium reveals the patient lived for several years after the operation</u>. Incidentally, Dodson also makes mention of a similar procedure being performed successfully during the 22nd Dynasty (c. 900 BCE). Academics maintain:

> *"The oldest known treatise on surgery . . . written in Egypt nearly 5,000 years ago, discloses to us the thoughts of the earliest man who reveals a scientific attitude of mind.*

Perception Vs. Reality

This treatise is therefore the earliest document in the history of science."[5]

---

[5] Ghalioungui, P., The House of Life Chp. 7, pp. 93 – 94 & Janssen, R., & Janssen, J., Growing Up in Ancient Egypt pp. 90 - 91 & Burn, A., & Selincourt, A., Herodotus: The Histories pp. 167 - 168 & Murphy, E., Diodorus on Egypt p. 35 & Muller, M., Mythology of All Races Vol. XII, p. 186 & Bunson, M., A Dictionary of Ancient Egypt p. 53 & Taton, R., History of Science p. 53 & Estes, J., The Medical Skills of Ancient Egypt p. 54 & Bucaille, M., Mummies of the Pharaohs pp. 102 - 103 & Hallowell, M., Herbal Healing pp. 161 - 162 & Butzer, C., Ancient Egypt: Discovering Its Splendors p. 120 & McGrew, R., Encyclopedia of Medical History p. 86 & Stetter, C., The Secret Medicine of the Pharaohs & Thornwald, J., Science and Secrets of Early Medicine p. 55 & Hall, M., The Secret Teachings of All Ages p. LXXIX & Muller, M., Mythology of All Races Vol. XII & Van Sertima, I., They Came Before Columbus p. 169 De Lubicz, R.A., The Temple in Man & Elephantine Museum: Artifact Collection & Dodson, A., Monarchs of the Nile p. 165 & Sedgewick, W., Tyler, H., & Bigelow, R., A Short History of Science p. 15 & Sadek, A., History of Medicine - Some Aspects of Medicine in Pharaonic Egypt (net) & Carlyon, R., Guide to the Gods p. 297

Due to racism and/or inadequate translation of the hieroglyphs, many negative characterizations have been made about ancient Egyptian medicine—some even characterizing it as ensorcellment. However, Sadek explains: *"Beside the names of over one hundred physicians from Pharaonic Egypt which were found in papyri, ostraca, stele, tombs, temples or on various personal objects (vases, rings etc.), our main sources on Ancient Egyptian Medicine . . . are the papyrus Smith, Ebers, Hearst, Kahoun, Berlin, Brooklyn, London, London-Leyde, Chester-Beatty, Carlsberg, Erman and Ramesseum. They include diagnosis and treatment of*

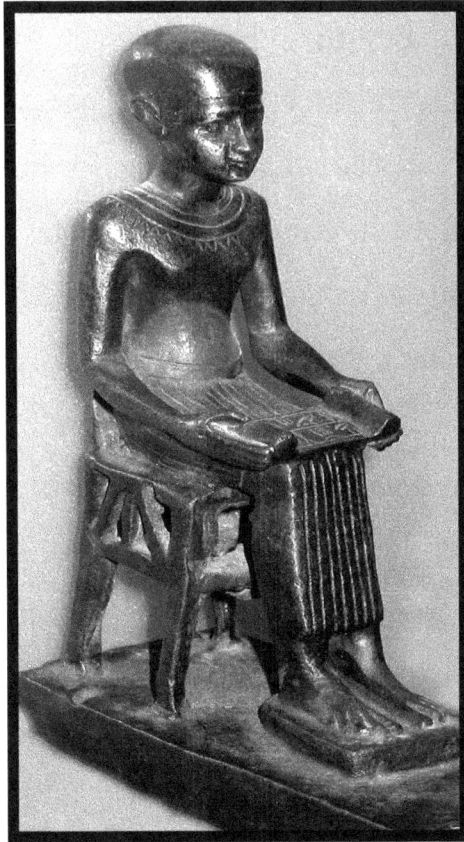

Imhotep

This is a statue of the ancient Egyptian physician Imhotep. He is reading a medical papyrus c. 2600 BCE. Widely acknowledged as a brilliant physician, architect, and vizier—Imhotep was later worshipped by the Greeks as *The God of Medicine.*

diseases and surgery as well as pharmacological receipts and formulas; some of them describe hopeless cases of illness and accidents, or deals with mental disturbances or spiritual problems (psychiatric and neurological cases) . . . we can find relatively few documents dealing with magical practices."

Perception Vs. Reality

I hope you've begun to grasp the fact that (*even in science*) Western perception does not always square with reality. Moreover, if the earlier case of Harvey were an isolated incident of medical laggardness, we might be able to dismiss the matter. However, with that premise too, failing to align with reality—to not delve deeper into the history of Western medicine would be unwise. After all, it is only demanding that we surrender our bodies (*or temples if you will*) to it from birth![6] Hence, deeper we shall go.

As previously mentioned, the empirical medical tradition in Northwestern Europe does not date back millenniums. No less important, nothing could be further from the truth than the notion that its origins were founded upon rational thought, hard scientific observation, and/or positive results!

---

[6] Bailey, R., <u>William Harvey - Father of Cardiovascular Medicine</u> & Horowitz, L., <u>Emerging Viruses and Vaccinations</u>
Unfortunately, infants are even being injected with problematic vaccines.

To quote Armstrong: *"Cardinal Richlieu was given horse-dung in wine [to drink] on his death-bed, and not by quacks but men we should nowadays call qualified doctors . . ."*[7]

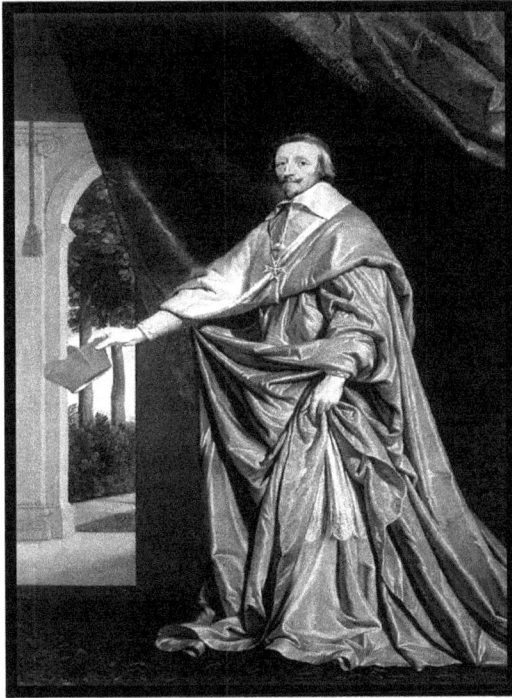

Cardinal-Duc de Richelieu

The Catholic Church of the Middle Ages oversaw the administration of the early medical tradition in Northwestern Europe. Cathedrals would serve as

---

[7] Armstrong, J., The Water of Life pp. 23 – 24

the region's first hospitals. Consequently, the views of the Vatican, *informed or otherwise*, controlled the course of medicine. As a matter of fact, the lengthy rejection of William Harvey's findings in blood circulation, were no doubt influenced by his medical opponents' loyalty and/or fear, of the Church's historical support for the (*metaphysical basis of disease*) views of the ancient Roman philosopher Galen. A number of Harvey's contemporaries openly declaring they would "*rather err with Galen than proclaim the truth with Harvey!*"[8]

With so little empirical medical understanding and training occurring in Medieval times, it is hardly surprising that the Church would eventually canonize the idea that bloodletting was the best way

---

[8] Schultz, S., William Harvey and the Circulation of the Blood: The Birth of a Scientific Revolution and Modern Physiology
Incredible admission considering such an "*err*" could cost someone their life! *Parenthetically, Energetic researchers are witnesses to the fact that some behavioral currents are not fazed by time.*

to treat many ailments. Accordingly, bloodletting was improperly prescribed for the following illnesses in Europe during the Middle Ages: nosebleeds, asthma, cholera, convulsions, epilepsy, gangrene, gout, indigestion, insanity, jaundice, leprosy, pneumonia, scurvy, smallpox, tuberculosis, and the list goes on.[9]

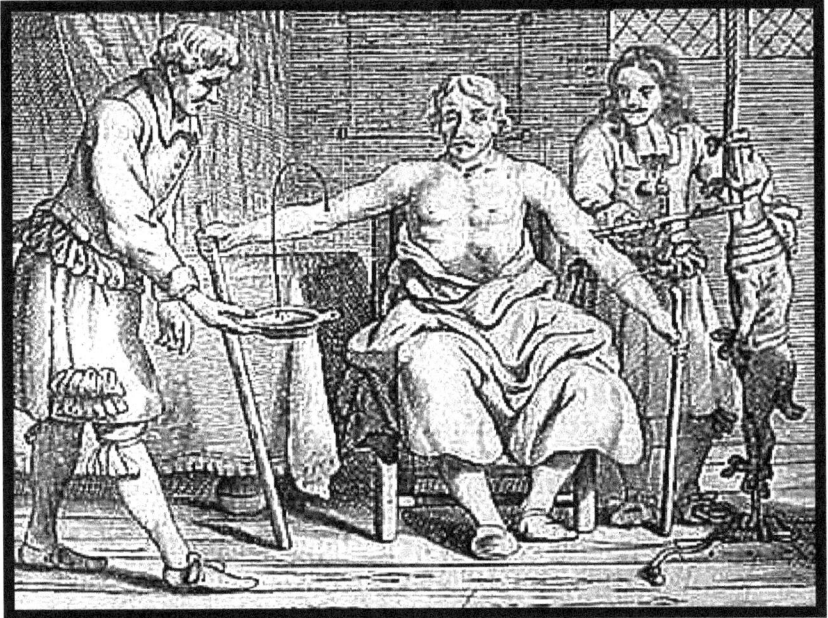

This patient is being bled and receiving a sheep's blood transfusion during the 17th century CE.

---

[9] Wikipedia: Bloodletting (net)
Incredibly, bloodletting was even performed on pregnant European women at the onset of labor.

Little wonder that for every decent medical outcome there were several that were not so agreeable. As the number of sick, bloody and dying people increased in the cathedrals—the Vatican decided that the clergy needed to get out of the unpleasant practice of bloodletting. In 1163, an edict by the Council of Tours prohibited the clergy from continuing to perform bloodletting. However, as Europe's formal physicians weren't thrilled about filling the void by becoming fulltime bloodletters, the Church relegated the untidy practice to Europe's barbers (*that's right—as in haircutters*).

The Church's 12th century edict gave state sanction for barbers to perform bloodletting and amputation in their shops. From that point, health problems that were unseen and inside the body (e.g., arthritis) were treated by physicians—those issues that were visible (e.g., a broken leg) by barbers. For so much as bloodletting and amputation were beneath the sensibilities of the average physician until 1744 CE, countless lives were entrusted to untrained, or regulated, barbershop owners for centuries . . .

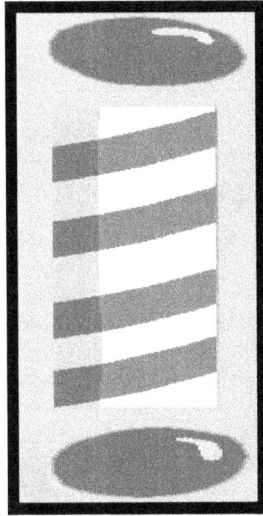

Red & White Barber Pole

Since most of us walk by symbols each day but have no understanding of their meaning, permit me to say a word here about today's barbershop pole. Dating to Medieval times, the red and white barber's pole was a very important sign.[10] It distinguished between a barber who performed bloodletting and one who did not. The color denotation was as

---

[10] Seigworth, G., <u>Bloodletting Over the Centuries</u> pp. 2022 - 2028

follows: red represents the blood being drawn from the arm; white represents the tourniquet (rag) that was tied around the arm to constrict the veins; while the pole itself represents the stick that was squeezed in the hand to dilate (enlarge) the veins before piercing and during the process (see page 13).[11]

In that bloodletting would remain a staple of European medicine until the late 1800s, of course, it came to North America with the 17th century colonists. Despite the fact that the outcomes of patients who underwent bloodletting in the colonies was no better than in Europe, there was no serious challenge to it before the 19th century on this side of the Atlantic either.

Upon reflection, I think it safe to conclude that the most notorious medical episode of bloodletting in America was the case of George Washington. In

---

[11] Seigworth, G., Bloodletting Over the Centuries pp. 2022-2028 & History of Barbering (net)

December of 1799, Washington caught a bad cold, which quickly turned into laryngitis and pneumonia. Three doctors were summoned to help the former president—*who was achy, feverous and could not swallow any medicine due to a very sore and swollen throat.* Unfortunately, Washington's doctors decided that the best course of treatment was to perform bloodletting on him. Over the next two days, Washington had five pints of blood withdrawn from his body—*even though his symptoms made it almost impossible to eat or drink anything.*

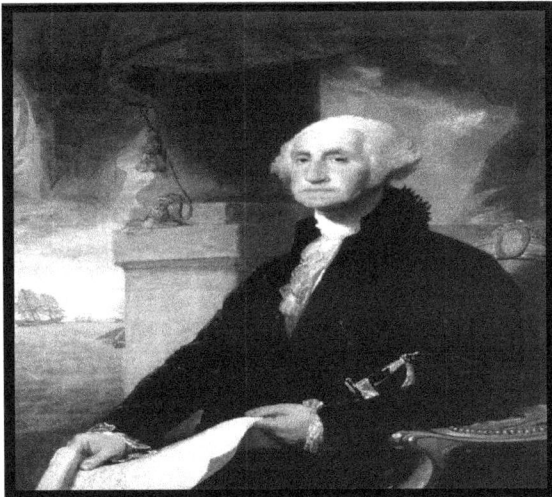

George Washington 1797

You don't have to be a rocket scientist to understand that losing five pints of blood in 48 hours could be problematic for someone who is healthy—let alone someone who's inflicted with laryngitis and pneumonia, and isn't capable of swallowing much liquid! Predictably, George Washington died on the evening of the second day of his ordeal.[12]

FYI: Today it is well established that *phlebotomy* (medical term for withdrawing or transfusing blood) is not an effective way to treat illness except when trying to adjust the body's red-blood cell count. Indeed, in most instances it can be harmful since it can weaken the patient, and make it more difficult for the body to fight infection. Hence, there really isn't any doubt that medically prescribing and performing bloodletting on the nation's first president played a crucial role in his death!

---

[12] Vadakan, V., A Physician Looks At The Death of George Washington (net)

As previously stated, the other Western medical procedure, unbelievably, carried out by barbers was amputation. European limbs were cut off hastily by barbers in barbershops for 600 years (*from the 1160s to 1740s*).   Having next to no medical training—barbers paid no attention to sanitation before, during, or after the procedure; and, because anesthesia was unknown—it was not uncommon for a patient to be brought in, held down, and after the amputation, have his open wound cauterized with little consideration being given to pain.

Atop all of this, while many amputations were warranted—many were not! For example, a limb could be amputated for simply being infected, fractured or broken as splinting and casting were still pretty unsophisticated. In passing, limbs could also be amputated for societal reasons; i.e., legal and/or Church sanctioned procedures. [13]

---

[13] Morton, D., 10 Excruciating Medical Treatments from the Middle Ages (net) &   Castiglioni, A., History of Medicine &

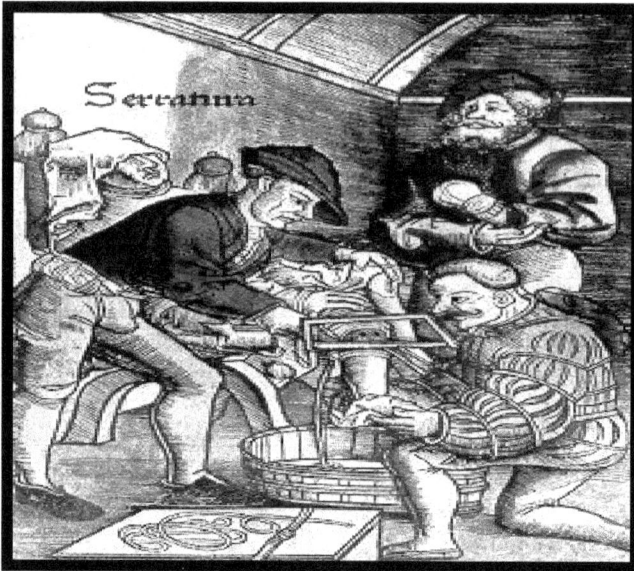

Portrait of amputation c. 1517 CE

Inasmuch as this sketch provides us with an honest

rendition of Medieval amputation—the fact that the

Bishop, M., The Horizon Book of the Middle Ages pp. 238, 244 - 246 & Cartwright, F., Disease and History pp. 54, 58 - 59 & Bloodletting, Encyclopedia of Medical History pp. 33 - 34 & Rogers, J.A., Sex and Race Vol. II, p. 398 & Zahoor, A., Hospitals and Medical Schools in the Dark and Middle Ages (net) & Himmelmann, L., From barber to surgeon- the process of professionalization pp. 69 - 87 & Peltier, L., Fractures: A History and Iconography of their Treatment & Wikipedia: Orthopedic Cast (net) & Adams, G., Doctors in Blue p. 133

The Church and the royals often used torture and brutality on the guilty, *and innocent*, in Inquisition Europe. At times, amputees were given a mixture of lettuce juice, the bile of a boar, briony, opium, henbane, hemlock juice, vinegar and wine before the procedure for pain; it was called *dwale*.

term *Sawbones* should become a common appellation for Northwestern Europe's barber-surgeons actually comes as no surprise.

Just as with bloodletting, the Western European medical practice of warranted, and unwarranted, amputation would follow the colonists to North America. The custom of the red and white barber pole would trail along as well. From the 1600s to the 1800s, amputation's role in American medicine would mirror that of its status in Europe. There was no serious questioning of amputation in American medicine until the Civil War.

In that amputation was a very common treatment for wounded soldiers, the war produced a high number of amputees on both sides. What's more, the patient outcomes were often poor: *about one out of every three amputees dying during, or soon after, the procedure*. The public (and soldiers) grew weary of years of this and eventually turned their frustration towards the war's surgeons—*widely referring to them as untrained and heartless butchers.* While it is true that the number of wounded was out of these doctors' hands, the countless number of poor outcomes from operating in blood and pus stained coats, with a single sponge, and undisinfected instruments **repeatedly**— leaves no doubt as to why these physicians should come to be characterized as *"untrained"* and *"heartless."*[14]

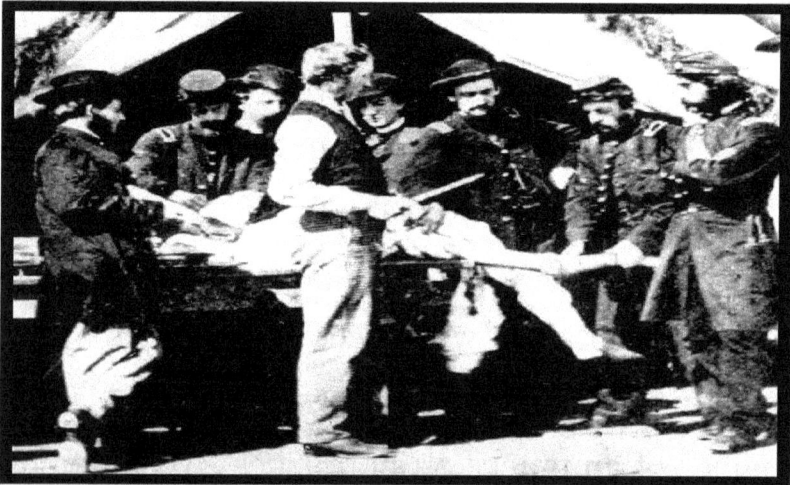

Doctor amputating leg at Gettysburg 1863

[14] Adams, G., <u>Doctors in Blue</u> & Goellnitz, J., <u>Civil War Surgery & Amputation</u> (net)
Many died of blood loss, gangrene, and blood poisoning after amputation. It must also be noted here that sponges were typically rinsed in cool bloody water and used over and over.

In closing, this chapter is entitled, <u>Perception Vs. Reality</u>. Despite the widespread modern perception, the reality is that many of Western medicine's early cardinal beliefs and practices were not just wrong—**they were extremely dangerous**! No less significant, the historical reality is physicians of the Old World had acquired a better grasp of the healing arts in several areas millenniums earlier![15]

According to Aristotle: *"He who thus considers things in their first growth and origin, whether a state or anything else, will obtain the clearest view of them."*[16] Western Europe's early medical perception that the heart pumped warm air, *not blood*, was wrong. Their stanch adherence to the medical practice of bloodletting was devastatingly

---

[15] Camp, J., <u>The Healer's Art: The Doctor through History</u> p. 27

In the words of Camp: *"With their ideas on drugs, on diet, and on a free health service for the poor, the doctors of Egypt and Mesopotamia seem to be much nearer our own time than do the barber-surgeons of the Middle Ages."*

[16] Ropes, L., <u>Aristotle</u> p. 248

wrong. Turning to amputation, not only was its application problematic—on top of that, it was poorly executed! Yet, even after an incalculable number of deaths and disastrous outcomes, the Western medical hierarchy would maintain and herald these faulty perceptions for centuries!

WHAT IF THE SAME WAY THEIR PERCEPTION WAS WRONG ABOUT DRINKING HORSE DUNG IN WINE

WHAT IF THE SAME WAY THEIR PERCEPTION WAS WRONG ABOUT HARVEY AND BLOOD CIRCULATION

WHAT IF THE SAME WAY THEIR PERCEPTION WAS WRONG ABOUT USING LEECHES TO PURIFY THE BODY

WHAT IF THE SAME WAY THEIR PERCEPTION WAS WRONG ABOUT BARBERSHOP AMPUTATION

WHAT IF THE SAME WAY THEIR PERCEPTION WAS DEAD WRONG ABOUT PERFORMING BLOODLETTING ON GEORGE WASHINGTON ON HIS DEATHBED

WHAT IF THE SAME WAY THEIR PERCEPTION WAS WRONG ABOUT REFUSING TO WASH THEIR HANDS AND INSTRUMENTS BEFORE TREATING PATIENTS

AND WHAT IF THE SAME WAY THE PERCEPTIONS OF DOCTORS WERE WRONG WHEN ENCOURAGING THEIR PATIENTS TO SMOKE CIGARETTES

ENERGETICS

Is the same way the medical hierarchy is wrong now about the realities of energetics?

Shocking Treatment Proposed For AIDS

Zapping the AIDS virus with low voltage electric current can nearly eliminate its ability to infect human white blood cells cultured in the laboratory, reports a research team at the Albert Einstein College of Medicine in New York City.

William D Lyman and his colleagues found arable to that produced by a cardiac pacemaker - reduced the infectivity of the AIDS virus (HIV) by 50 to 95 percent. Their experiments, described March 14 [1991] in Washington D.C., at the First International Symposium on Combination Therapies, showed that the shocked viruses lost the ability to make an enzyme crucial to their reproduction, and could no longer cause the white cells to clump together - two key signs of virus infection.

The finding could lead to tests of implantable electrical devices or dialysis-like blood treatments in HIV-infected patients Lyman says. In addition, he suggests that blood banks might use electricity to zap HIV, and vaccine developers might use electrically incapacitated viruses as the basis for an AIDS vaccine.

Science News, Vol. 139 No. 13, (Mar. 30, 1991), p. 207

Scientists say electric current may help fight AIDS

REUTER NEWS SERVICE

NEW YORK — Doctors at a prestigious New York medical center are testing a new way to fight AIDS — using electrical energy to weaken the killer virus — and say their first results are encouraging.

Researchers William Lyman and Steven Kaali of the Albert Einstein School of Medicine said Tuesday that initial laboratory tests have shown electrical current can weaken the virus believed to cause acquired immune deficiency syndrome.

The two men said they plan to move to the next phase of the experiment in April using blood samples from people with AIDS.

If their tests are successful, the researchers hope it could lead to a new way to treat AIDS patients, possibly involving a dialysis-type machine in which an AIDS patient's blood would be treated with electrical current outside the body.

"What we have done is expose the AIDS virus in laboratory circumstances to electrical current and then incubated the virus with white blood cells susceptible to the virus. We found that the virus became much more ineffective," Kaali, a specialist in the medical use of electrical current, said.

Lyman, an AIDS researcher and associate professor of pathology at Einstein, likened the new technique to chemotherapy.

"You are not going to get rid of the tumor, but you could get rid of enough of it to help the patient lead a normal life. This is not a cure but a new tool," Lyman said.

He added that the use of electrical energy has no toxic side effects and that a similar technique has been used as a treatment for reducing herpes.

Houston Post, Wednesday, March 20, 1991 A-10

It is not a character flaw to make a mistake; however, to refuse to acknowledge and correct an error once its been brought to the fore, is an entirely different matter . . .

WARNING:
The Use of Allopathic Medicine may be hazardous to your Health

Warning:
The use of Allopathic Medicine may be hazardous to your Health

The term that is most commonly used to designate the current model of conventional medicine in America is *Allopathic*. First coined by Dr. Samuel Hahnemann in the 1840s, the label stems from two Greek words: *allos* which means "other" and *pathos* which means "suffering." Hahnemann chose this term to emphasize the fact that Western medicine was mainly focused upon the symptoms of an illness, as opposed to its cause. The glaring problems with this approach are threefold: first, it is restrictive; second, it does little to fight, or ward off, disease; and third, the side-effects from prolonged symptom management can become worst than the primary illness itself!

Being trained and practiced in the conventional Western medicine of his day, Dr. Hahnemann's skepticism was well-founded. *As a young physician it soon became clear to him that the drugs he prescribed seldom led to healing—and everyone who had surgery was at risk during, and after, the trauma of an operation to other kinds of suffering!*

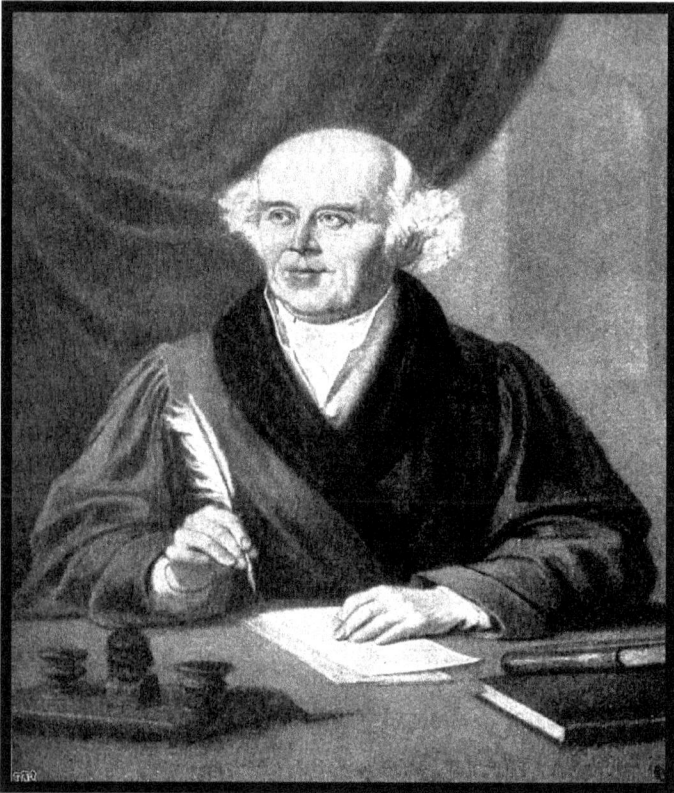

Christian Friedrich Samuel Hahnemann

Hence, his early departure from the discipline and subsequent reassessment of Western medicine as being far more **allopathic** in nature than **healing**.[1]

---

[1] Hahnemann held his conviction so strongly that he broke from convention to initiate a new approach to the treatment of illness. In 1796, he established the *Homeopathic* theory, and practice, of medicine in Europe.

Warning:
The use of Allopathic Medicine may be hazardous to your Health

Today, there are a number of conventionally trained physicians who object to the allopathic designation being applied to their profession. However, with the foundations of American medicine being dead set, *and financially pivoting*, upon treating illness with powerful side-effect producing drugs and/or cutting the body open—Hahnemann's basic assessment and warnings have no less merit today than they did one-hundred and sixty years ago. In fact, I am at a loss to tally the number of people I've encountered who explain that once they begin treatment for one illness—other health concerns crop up.[2]

---

[2] To evaluate a system, you can't just listen to its administrators or staff—you have to talk to its clientele; **that is what I have been doing for the past two years**! From botched medical procedures, to hospital inflections, to drug side-effects—*the solution to one health issue creating some other problem has often been expressed.* Watching a hospital visit on TV and experiencing one in real life are two wholly different matters! For instance, I recently spoke to a woman who contracted colitis (infected colon) shortly after having some dental work done. After being admitted to the hospital, the antibiotics she was given changed her potassium levels such that her muscles and joints began to trouble her. While trying to rectify that problem, she caught hospital pneumonia. Ultimately, it was several weeks (and thousands of dollars later) before she was actually able to return home.

Despite the constant media drumbeat about the *"Wonders of American Medicine,"* the facts are we pay more for health care (per capita) than the citizens of any other nation; however, our health outcomes do not measure up in many important areas. Indeed, *save expenditures*, America's health care rankings are pedestrian across the board. Here is the bottom line: *Although America spends more on health care than any other nation, the life expectancy of Americans isn't even in the top-twenty: it is an underwhelming forty-seventh!*[3]

Truth be told, allopathic medicine has caused a significant amount of, *fiscal and physical,* pain in America. **Two independent peer reviewed studies, headed by Dr. Gary Null and Dr. Barbara Starfield, have concluded that one**

---

[3] Geyman, J., Health Care in America: Can Our Ailing System Be Healed? & World Development Indicators 2002: Health Statistics (CD) & NationMaster: Health Statistics (net) & CIA World Factbook: Life Expectancy 18 December 2003 to 18 December 2008 (net) & World Health Organization: Health Statistics 2010

**of the leading causes of death in America, is
the nation's health care system itself!**[4]
Astonishingly, these researchers found that
anywhere from 18,000 to 60,000 Americans die
each month from one of the following causes:
*unnecessary surgeries; medical staff errors;
infections contracted in hospitals; outpatient care;
and, from FDA approved medications (drugs) that
were administered precisely as prescribed!*[5]

What a fickle society: I say this because we all
experienced the relentless fervor of the corporate
media after September 11th and the tragic loss of
nearly 3,000 Americans lives. Of course, that
emotionalism was understandable and even to be

---

[4] The industry term for unnecessary death is *iatrogenic:* i.e.,
death accidentally caused by a medical professional.
[5] Starfield, B., Is US Health Really the Best in the World?
JAMA Vol. 284, No. 4, July 26, 2000 pp. 483-485 & Null,
G., & Dean, C., & Feldmen, M., & Rasio, D., & Smith, D.,
Death By Medicine (net) & Horowitz, L., Emerging Viruses
and Vaccinations & Eustace Mullins, Murder by injection
These figures do not include annual deaths caused by FDA
approved vaccinations (see page 201).

expected. However, what's not so easy to understand is how does the same media herald an industry that causes more than 700,000 needless deaths each year? Or, turn a blind eye towards political figures who swear to protect the public, yet routinely take steps that don't merely fail to make us safer—but guarantee us more of the same?

Believe it or not, I am not someone who wants to slam doctors, nurses or any other health care professional; <u>no doubt many of them are capable, moral and compassionate people</u>. Even more, if you get into a serious accident—**you had better get to an emergency room stat**—and pray that one of the afore mentioned is there waiting for you: *physical trauma can be a very serious matter!!!*

However, the fundamental disconnect between corporate health and human health is causing real harm! Just one quick for instance: in his <u>Death by Medicine</u>, Null explains that well over 7 million unnecessary surgeries are performed in America each year. <u>That's over 19,000 surgeries a day—and many of these are performed on vulnerable women</u>. Of course, the cost a single surgery can run into the tens of thousands of dollars. Put bluntly:

> *"American physicians are generally way too eager to use the surgeon's knife to carve up and chop out whatever they think is ailing you, at great expense to you and great profit to them and the hospitals they work for . . ."*[6]

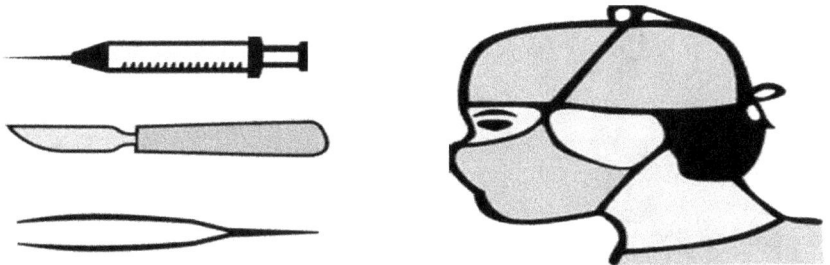

---

[6] Rondberg, T., <u>Under the Influence of Modern Medicine</u> & Mindell, E., & Hopkins, V., <u>Prescription Alternatives</u>
I just met a woman who was diagnosed with Crohn's disease years ago. The prescribed treatment was to cut the infected intestine out. Today, after several surgeries, she still has Crohn's—but now with other medical issues from having too few intestines. Two other women I know face serious, *and life altering*, issues from gastric bypass surgery (the removal of most of the stomach for weight loss). Outcomes like this compel us to reconsider the application of surgical medicine, and its Medieval amputative genesis (see pages 19 – 23).

Look, we are at a kind of precipice (*and some of us more than others*). <u>The quick diagnosis:</u> A fiscally challenged nation hemorrhaging money in the area of health care; mediocre outcomes for many of those with access; health care workers who are stretched from both ends; no shortage of greedy executives; no bold political, or regulatory, figures who are willing to put human health above that of corporations; and a restrictive approach to medical treatment—all lead to a prognosis that is negative.

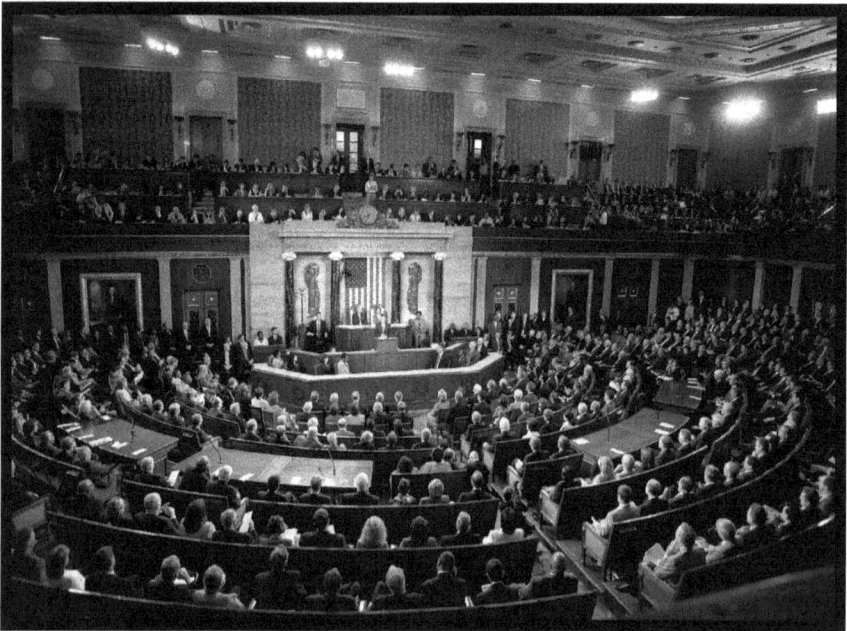

Obama Health Care Speech before 111th Congress

*To wait for those to save you who are paid rather handsomely not to is insane. You can cross your fingers and hope that the current health care system will not fail you, or you can do what Bob Beck was so quick to advise—**You Can Take Back Your Power**! Should you choose the latter, I simply ask that you consider all of the information in this book with an open mind. **I did, and an incurable disease** (according to the CDC and medical establishment) **which plagued me for decades is no longer an issue in my life!***

The Medical Industrial Complex

Before the turn of the 20th century, a good deal of the American public believed in homeopathic medicine. This approach was often based upon natural and inexpensive cures that were administered in the home. Many of these cures were, and still are, effective. For instance, drinking cabbage juice for stomach ulcers is one example of a proven homeopathic/holistic remedy.[1]

During the last half of the 19th century, a businessman named John D. Rockefeller would come to dominate America's oil industry. Through innovation, under-pricing, buying out his competition, and bribery—Rockefeller's Standard Oil came to control 90% of the petroleum (oil) produced in America.[2] To be brief, Standard Oil's extreme wealth and domination over the industry

---

[1] Carper, J., Food Your Miracle Medicine & Giller, R., Natural Prescriptions: Dr. Giller's Natural Treatments & Vitamin Therapies For Over 100 Common Ailments
The allopathic treatment for stomach ulcers frequently calls for antibiotics, which can be risky (see page 29).
[2] The driving force for crude wasn't the car—it was kerosene.

caused great national consternation; eventually leading to anti-trust court decisions against the company just after the turn of the 20th century.

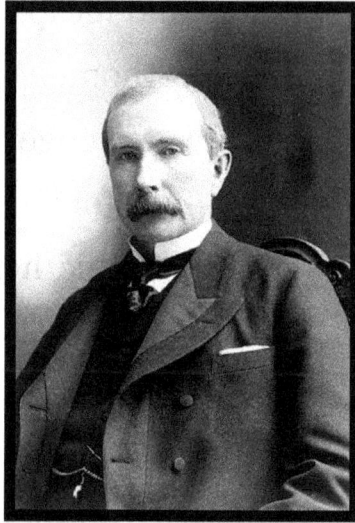

John D. Rockefeller 1885

You've heard the expression *"Nice guys finish last."* Well, the fact that Rockefeller was, by all measure, the wealthiest businessman in America by far, speaks volumes. Despite giving great sums away as a philanthropist, Rockefeller was an industrialist who ignored calls for worker safety in coal mines; he opposed the eight hour work day; he opposed child labor laws; he believed a less educated public was good for the business class (*ignorant people often being less confrontational*); and he even testified that had he been able to stop men in his employ from causing the deaths of 19 striking coal miners during the Ludlow Massacre—***he would not!***[3]

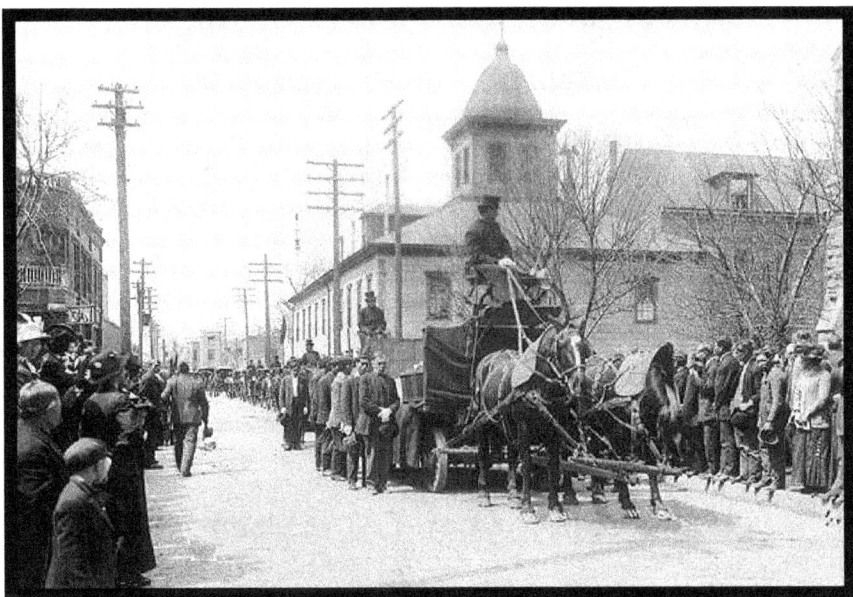

Funeral for Ludlow Coal Strikers 1914

One of the petro-chemical divisions of Standard Oil produced medicinal drugs. Mullins points out that

---

[3] Gage, B., The Day Wall Street Exploded p. 94 & Zinn, H., A People's History of the United States pp. 346 – 349 & Wikipedia: Ludlow Massacre (net) & Horowitz, L., The Red Double Cross (net)

the family's involvement with medicates dated back to John's father, William, who sold crude oil to people as an erroneous cure for cancer in the 1800s. In the words of Eustace Mullins:

> *"William Rockefeller had become an oil entrepreneur after salt wells at Tarentum, near Pittsburgh, were discovered in 1842 to be flowing with oil. The owner . . . Samuel L. Kier, began to bottle the oil and sell it for medicinal purposes. One of his earliest wholesalers was William Rockefeller. The 'medicine' was originally labeled 'Kier's Magic Oil'. Rockefeller printed his own labels, using 'Rock Oil' or 'Seneca Oil' . . . Rockefeller achieved his greatest notoriety and his greatest profits by advertising himself as 'William Rockefeller, the Celebrated Cancer Specialist.'"*[4]

---

[4] Mullins, E., <u>Murder by Injection</u> Chp. 10
With large mark-up and low overhead, Rockefeller made a lot of money selling his cancer cure across America. He was one of the nation's many 19th century snake-oil salesmen.

As for the son, John's industrial production of medicates fueled his desire to increase the public demand. What's more, *old habits being hard to break*, the business strategy of doing whatever it took to gain complete control over a market would accompany his aim—usher in **The Flexner Report**.

In that I've never heard the beginnings of the Medical Industrial Complex (MIC) discussed more eloquently, allow me to defer to Dr. Len Horowitz:

> *"During this time, John D. Rockefeller and his associates were making a concerted effort to control the entire field of medicine in America. During the 1890s, Rockefeller interests in medical education and 'scientific medicine' were spearheaded by Frederick T. Gates, John D. Rockefeller's investment manager. 1901 saw the founding of the Rockefeller Institute for Medical Research ... In 1904, the Cold Spring Harbor Laboratory (home to today's Human Genome Project)*

was built on the estates of John Foster and Allen Dulles, lawyers for the Rockefeller Standard Oil Company . . . By 1907, medical education had been mostly monopolized by the Rockefeller consortium . . . Through Rockefeller cohorts in the Andrew Carnegie Endowment for the Advancement of Teaching, Abraham Flexner was appointed to survey medical schools throughout America. This led to the infamous 'Flexner Report' that vilified every alternative to drug-based medicine . . . Rockefeller's political control over this American medical coup was clearly reflected in Flexner family relations. Abraham Flexner served on the Rockefellers General Education Board. Abraham Flexner's brother, Simon, headed the Rockefeller Institute of Medical Research. Simon's brother, Bernard, later joined the board of trustees of the Rockefeller Foundation after he helped found the politically powerful Council on Foreign Relations . . ."[5]

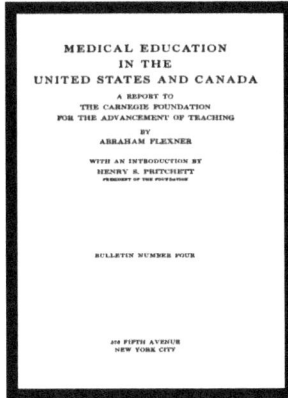

MEDICAL EDUCATION
IN THE
UNITED STATES AND CANADA
A REPORT TO
THE CARNEGIE FOUNDATION
FOR THE ADVANCEMENT OF TEACHING
BY
ABRAHAM FLEXNER

WITH AN INTRODUCTION BY
HENRY S. PRITCHETT
PRESIDENT OF THE FOUNDATION

BULLETIN NUMBER FOUR

576 FIFTH AVENUE
NEW YORK CITY

Under the auspices of wanting to improve the health and education of the medical community in America, Abraham Flexner would turn American health care into an allopathic cherry—ripe for Rockefeller's picking! Many sweeping medical changes were proposed in the nearly 400 page report; however, allow me to touch upon some of the most tectonic: (1) it called for much stricter

---

[5] Horowitz, L. Dr., The American Red Double-cross (net) & Becker, R., & Seldon, G., The Body Electric p. 82 & Sullivan, D., A Short History of Eugenics (PDF)
Rockefeller also funded eugenics research (see page 188). By the 1940s, tens of thousands of Americans had been victimized by the nation's compulsory sterilization laws.

regulation and government control over hospitals and physicians; (2) it called for the fees of American Medical Association (AMA) sanctioned training to be raised; (3) it recommended closing many medical schools (*including the leading African-American medical colleges*); (4) it encouraged doctors to charge the poor the same prices for treatment as the rich (*before this doctors often charged patients according to their means*); and (5), it denigrated those forms of inexpensive treatment which weren't considered **scientific enough**: i.e., osteopathic (musculoskeletal) eclectic (natural herbs) physiomedicalism (vital force) naturopathy (natural self-healing) homeopathic (serial diluted medicates) and last but not least—electrotherapeutics.

With the American Medical Association's full public support, *and Rockefeller's deal making beneath the surface*, Flexner's recommendations were enacted straightaway. The effects upon medicine were swift and clear: (1) within eight years, the number of medical schools in the nation went from 650 to 50; (2) every African American medical college was closed; (3) those medical colleges which taught alternative medicine were not given an accreditation by the AMA, so they eventually closed; (4) this all led to a reduction in the number of doctors, which effected availability and pricing; and (5), insomuch as there was very little federal legislation over medical treatments before the 1900s—the report's canonization of treating illness with drugs and/or surgery, was Rockefeller's coup de gras: _the fusion between industrial medicates and U.S. health care_.

This period represents the wholesale entrenchment of allopathic medicine in America. It was also the beginning of big hospitals with long patient stays; increased drug sales for pain; increased drug sales for disease; and an increase in surgery—with fees arbitrarily being set and raised. Because this approach to healing was incredibly expensive (_much higher than ever before_) health insurance and big charities weren't created to make sure that every patient got the best possible care—*but to make sure that the medical industry didn't collapse on itself!*

Today, pharmaceuticals play a critical role in U.S. medicine. Just about every illness has a manufactured drug that's prescribed for it by an allopathic physician. While some of these drugs are effective, many are not (*with a number causing real harm*). Despite this, pharmaceuticals generate huge profits for drug companies. <u>Although the American public represents about 5% of the world's population—we consume about 50% of all of the pharmaceuticals sold worldwide; a fact that is a direct consequence of the report created by Rockefeller lackey Abraham Flexner</u>. According to Mullins:

> *"The Rockefellers control every one of the largest drug companies in the world. When I say control—I mean directly . . . Among the boards of directors and officials of each of the 18 largest drug companies in the world, they*

have men from Chase Manhattan Bank, from the Exxon oil company, and so forth . . . With this kind of control, and the [health care] monopoly, they have been jacking up the health cost on the American people monthly—not yearly, but monthly . . ."[6]

Another big-ticket item in MIC medicine is cancer treatment. Bob Beck explains that the cost of treatment for the average cancer patient is well over 350,000 dollars.[7] It's rather remarkable that on the one hand, physicians tell you that cancer has no cure (*not that their methods may not cure you—but that there is no cure*); then they cut you open; they remove parts of your body; they flood every cell in your body with toxic chemicals (*which make you*

---

[6] <u>Prescription for Disaster</u> Dvd & Bobby Lee Show: <u>Murder by Injection Interview E. Mullins</u> Dvd
Truth be told, there are more drug company lobbyists than there are members of Congress. For AMA mission and Big Pharma profits, see pages 185 and 192 – 194.
[7] One can't help but be reminded of the jibe, *"More people make their living off cancer, than actually have the disease."*

miserable for weeks); then, they bathe your body in radiation (*which has long been known to jeopardize, not promote, health*). After his mother underwent conventional cancer treatment, a prominent doctor would characterize her experience thus: <u>butchering</u>, <u>poisoning</u>, *and* <u>cooking</u>. To quote Mendelsohn: *"Modern cancer surgery someday will be regarded with the same kind of horror that we now regard the use of leeches in George Washington's time."*[8]

America spends more for health care than any other nation. This pie represents the entire American economy (over 14 trillion dollars). The pie slice (HC) represents the amount spent on health care (2.5 trillion) and it continues to rise.

---

[8] Global Sciences Congress: <u>THE BOB BECK INTERVIEW</u> & Lynes, B., <u>Cancer Solutions: Rife, Energy Medicine and Medical Politics</u> & Mullins, E., <u>Murder by Injection</u>
Once more, the side-effects for those who survive can be life altering. For example, I recently met a woman who underwent conventional cancer therapy. While it appears that her cancer has been controlled for now—the treatment damaged her heart so seriously that she has also had to undergo heart surgery to have a pacemaker implanted.

The World Health Organization's ranking of the world's health systems

1	France	21	Belgium
2	Italy	22	Colombia
3	San Marino	23	Sweden
4	Andorra	24	Cyprus
5	Malta	25	Germany
6	Singapore	26	Saudi Arabia
7	Spain	27	United Arab Emirates
8	Oman	28	Israel
9	Austria	29	Morocco
10	Japan	30	Canada
11	Norway	31	Finland
12	Portugal	32	Australia
13	Monaco	33	Chile
14	Greece	34	Denmark
15	Iceland	35	Dominica
16	Luxembourg	36	Costa Rica
17	Netherlands	37	United States of ***America***
18	United Kingdom		
19	Ireland	38	Slovenia
20	Switzerland		

What does this all mean? It means that at the turn of the 20th century, health options and freedoms were taken away from the individual and given to businessmen. The obvious problem with this is the principal concern of businessmen is _fiscal_, rather than _physical_, wellbeing! No less disconcerting, as long as there is big money in health care—_we are creating a financial incentive for people to be sick._[9]

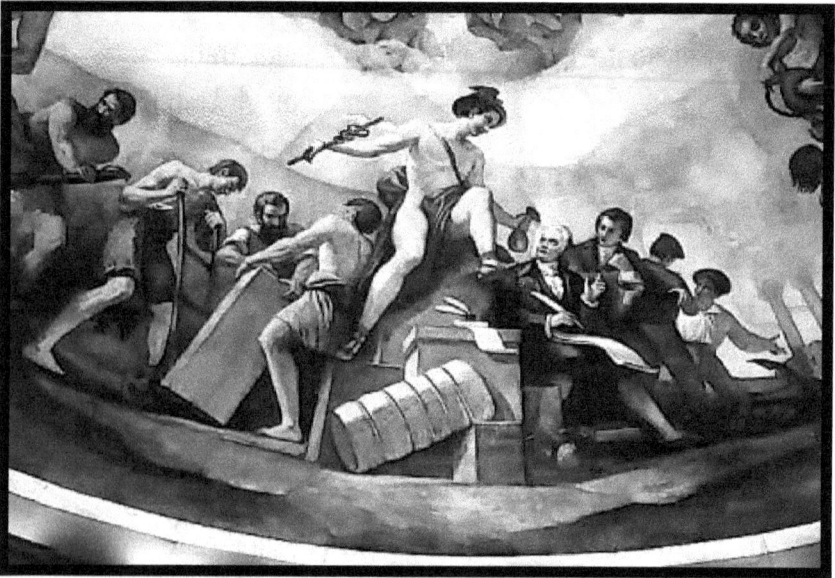

The Apotheosis in the Washington Capitol

---

[9] Carter, J., Racketeering in Medicine: The Suppression of Alternatives & Sicko DVD
With pitchmen and lobbyists everywhere, little wonder Carter asserts: _"Corporations now control the practice of medicine."_

ENERGETICS

The Apotheosis is a tremendous fresco that was painted by the Greek-Italian artist Constantino Brumidi in tribute to George Washington. It is positioned so as to be seen through the oculus of the dome in the rotunda of the American Capitol. The scene depicts Mercury (God of Commerce) paying off a lawmaker (politician). The stick in his hand, with the two serpents intertwined around it, is known as the *Caduceus*. From ancient times, the Caduceus has been seen as the symbol of merchants, gamblers, liars and thieves. It is noteworthy that the first symbol of the American Medical Association, and several other health organizations, was the Caduceus.[10]

Symbology is how the elite hide in plain sight. However, the 21st century is requiring us all to grasp

---

[10] Henry, W., & Gray, M., Freedom's Gate & New World Encyclopedia: Caduceus (net) & Wikipedia: Apotheosis (net)
The term *Apotheosis* means, "deification." It is said that the painting is considered to represent Washington's Masonic ascension to divinity.

the fact that there is a vast difference between the meanings of *The Rod of Imhotep* and the *Caduceus*—the former <u>health</u>, the latter <u>commerce</u>. Let me leave you with this valuation of the Medical Industrial Complex by Dr. Robert Mendelson:

> *"I no longer believe in modern medicine. I believe that despite all the super technology and elite bedside manner that's supposed to make you feel about as well cared for as an astronaut on the way to the moon—the greatest danger to your health is the doctor who practices modern medicine. I believe that modern medicine's treatments for disease are seldom effective, and that they're often more dangerous than the disease they're designed to treat . . . The dangers are compounded by the widespread use of dangerous procedures for non-diseases . . . More than ninety percent of modern medicine could disappear from the face of the earth—doctors, hospitals, drugs, and*

equipment—and the effect on our health would be immediate and beneficial . . . Modern medicine has gone too far, by using in everyday situations extreme treatments designed for critical conditions . . . So, when you go to the doctor, you're seen not as a person who needs help with his or her health, but as a potential market for the medical factory's products . . ."[11]

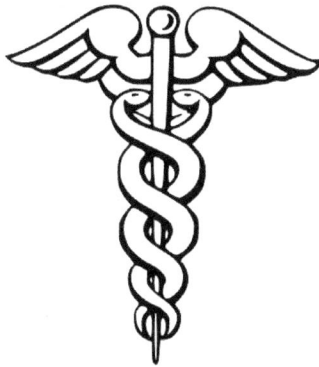

---

[11] Mendelsohn, R., <u>Confessions of a Medical heretic</u> pp. 12 – 13

There is a rudimentary disconnect between the mental constructs of a healer and a mechanic. The latter is a part exchanger, simply searching for some device or/and additive to create *"better performance,"* which makes genuine health nothing more than an afterthought! But the former understands that most of us were given everything we need to be at our optimum; thus, focusing on maintaining and/or restoring the natural balance. FYI: <u>Energetics rests with the latter.</u>

Who Is This Bob Beck?

My introduction to Bob Beck and Energetics did not occur until 2007. At first blush, *as is so often the case with exceptional souls*, my impression was similar to the Corinthians' view of Paul—*His words are weighty and powerful, but his bodily presence is weak!* In reflection, his presentation was to be expected; he was a senior who had overcome several health challenges in his life. Again however, just as with Paul—*his heart and deeds were equal to his words!*

Robert C. Beck, D.Sc. was born in 1925 and he died in 2002. During his life he would achieve a great deal as a scientist and inventor. Professionally, Beck was an engineer, U.C. professor, physicist and consultant to the United States Navy (*actually performing classified project work for the nation*).

Like many Americans, Beck's health began to deteriorate in his middle years. But receiving little relief from conventional medicine, he began to turn his attention, *and scientific training*, to the field of Energy Medicine. His first company developed an electroencephalograph, which led to extensive research on the electrical properties of the brain. Eventually, Beck invented a brain-tuning device which helps to alleviate anxiety, addictions, insomnia and depression—by using frequencies to help rejuvenate, heal and restimulate the brain's neurotransmitters! Later, he tested electrical frequencies on the lymphatic system because many viral agents settled there. He also developed a pulse generator to supply electromagnetic energy to specific parts of the body.

By the 1980s, Beck had investigated many therapeutic uses for electromagnetic energy. But in the early 1990s, Beck learned about an exciting discovery by Steven Kaali and William Lyman. These doctors found that when the Human Immunodeficiency Virus (HIV) was exposed to a very small electrical charge—its protein walls were damaged to such an extent that the virus was no longer a serious threat to the body![1]   These researchers surmised that through a process of dialysis (*pulling the blood out of the body, pumping it past electrodes, and then returning it*) patients with HIV would be helped. Their view was that it should only take about fifteen years to perfect the medical process for humans.[2]

Finding Kaali and Lyman's fifteen year forecast completely unreasonable—Beck went to work. His many years of research in low-level electrical fields and energy medicine would make him the perfect man for the job. In a short time, Beck had not only performed successful blood electrification—he was doing it safely without any need for dialysis at all! <u>Because of Bob Beck's work, many people with AIDS, Prostate Cancer, Lyme Disease, Rheumatoid</u>

---

[1] See page 25.

[2] By the by, it's been fifteen years—and not a peep by the MIC about the recognized promise of blood electrification against HIV or other illnesses. *I wonder why that is . . .*

Arthritis, Herpes B, Chronic Fatigue Immune Dysfunction Syndrome, Hepatitis A and B, Cervical Cancer, and Lupus—no longer have any symptoms of these diseases!!![3]

You'd think these achievements would have made Beck a CNN and Oprah regular, but instead it made him Establishment Enemy Number One. At 3:00 one morning, FDA agents raided Bob Beck's home with guns drawn! They jostled and threatened to lock him up if he didn't stop helping people. The two things that saved Beck was he wasn't charging people; and, consenting adults still have a legal right to volunteer for research projects. Despite being marginalized in the United States, health professions in Mexico would nominate Dr. Robert C. Beck, D.Sc. for the Nobel Peace Prize in Medicine,

---

[3] These research subjects' blood was analyzed with dark field microscopy, before and after, electrification. What is more, medical professionals reviewed and verified all of Beck's findings! It should also be noted that of the hundreds of people Beck worked with—not one has ever accused him of harming them or sued him in a court of law!

for his well-documented medical accomplishments![4]

Look, as incredible as this all sounds, **it's all true.** While Beck was clearly no philosopher, biblical scholar or historian—and I most certainly disagree with his use of the term *Immortal Blood*, as nothing in this temporal plane will last forever—what he was, was a man who believed in <u>Right</u> and <u>Wrong</u>. Equally laudable, as a slave to astute observation and quantifiable outcomes after regimented experimentation—he never placed money over empirical truth; *for both, I applaud him!* Over a thousand years ago, Confucius taught: *"The scholarly man who places personal comfort over truth, is not worthy of his title."* It is manifest that he was not talking about **Robert C. Beck**, as he was a man who was clearly deserving of the nomenclature—**Doctor of Science**![5]

---

[4] As those inside the tent seldom wish to acknowledge the work of those on the outside, *though warranted*, Beck's nomination received little attention from Nobel voters.
[5] <u>The medical establishment could not buy, or scare, him off</u>!

Bob Beck Lecture: Take Back Your Power

Researchers

BOB BECK LECTURE

TAKE BACK YOUR POWER!

CONQUERING "INCURABLES" WITH MICROCURRENTS!

BLOOD ELECTRIFICATION is a proven, startling, rapid, inexpensive and safe discovery for proven remissions.

A suppressed medical breakthrough now apparently guarantees anyone total power to reverse previously "incurable" diseases *INCLUDING HIV and CANCER* with a simple electronic device.

A tested, revolutionary but almost unbelievable medical discovery may enable rapid AIDS, Epstein-Barr, Hepatitis, Cancer, Lupus and other disease elimination. Total cost is about $1.32 per patient per remission of symptoms and requires NO doctors, surgery, drugs, diet, medical bills, shots, herbs, or outside intervention. This breakthrough is now *yours* despite apparent suppression by medical and pharmaceutical cartels.

Workshop

EVERYTHING needed to enable rapid do-it-yourself recoveries from previously "incurable" viruses, backeria, microbes, pathogens, fungi, and parasites in TOTAL PRIVACY with complete instructions plus legal loopholes which may keep researchers unmolested by FDA while healing themselves and others. *Most subjects are symptom free within 4 weeks.*

Developed independently by Bob Beck, it's here NOW !

We have nothing for sale!

A PROPOSED EXPERIMENTAL/THEORETICAL, NONINVASIVE, NONPHARMACEUTICAL, IN VIVO METHOD FOR RAPID NEUTRALIZATION OF HIV VIRUS IN HUMAN SUBJECTS.

Revision March 20, 1997. Copyright © 1991/1997 by Robert C. Beck, D.Sc.

In a remarkable discovery at Albert Einstein College of Medicine, NYC in 1990, it was shown that a minute current (50 to 100 *micro* amperes) can alter outer protein layers of HIV virus in a petri dish so as to prevent its later attachment to receptor sites. (Science News, March 30, 1991 pg. 207.) It may also reverse Epstein-Barr (chronic fatigue syndrome), hepatitis, and herpes B. HIV-positive users of this enclosed information may expect a *NEGATIVE* PCR test (no more HIV detectable in blood) after 30 days. This is reminiscent of a well proven cure for snakebite by application of electric current that instantly neutralizes the venom's toxicity. (Lancet, July 26, 1986, pg. 229.) And there may be several other as yet undiscovered or untested viruses neutralizable with this discovery, perhaps more surprisingly, even the common cold.

This very simple and valid blood clearing treatment offered great promise as a positive method for immobilizing known strains of HIV still present and contaminating some European and US blood bank reserve supplies. It was further suggested that infected human HIV carriers could be cured by removing their blood, treating it electrically and returning it by methods similar to dialysis as described in US patent # 5, 188,738. Dr. S. Kaali, MD, projected that "years of testing will be in order before such an *in vitro* (blood removed for treatment) device can be made ready for widespread use" (Longevity, Dec 1992, pg. 14.) This paper reveals an alternate "do-it-yourself" approach for electrifying/purifying blood *with no dialysis, implants, or medical intervention*.

In the writer's opinion both blood and lymph can be cleared *in vivo* (which means blood isn't removed or skin ever penetrated) simply, rapidly, and inexpensively with similar but *non-invasive* techniques described herein. All are fully disclosed in this paper. Also included is the proven schematic, parts lists, electrode construction and and complete instructions. Electronic and controlled electroporation approaches may well make vaccines (even if possible someday), pharmaceuticals, supplements, herbs, and diet therapies, plus other proposed remedies obsolete, even if they worked and were universally available at no cost.

In a public lecture (Oct. 19, 1991) the writer proposed this theoretical do-it-yourself method for accomplishing HIV, parasite, fungal, viral and pathogen 'neutralization' *in vivo*. Subsequently, his original modalities and protocols have been extensively peer reviewed, refined, simplified and made universally affordable (under $75 for *both* devices including batteries when self-made). These two simple treatments used in tandem can potentially nullify well over 95% (and perhaps 100%) of known HIV strains residing in *both* blood, lymph, and other body tissue and fluids. Following is a summary of several years of offshore feedback with this noniatrogenic, do-it-yourself, simple and inexpensive experimental solution to the ever escalating AIDS dilemma. There are no known side effects since milliampere currents are much lower than those in FDA approved TENS, CES and muscle stimulators which have been in daily use for many years. Battery replacement costs are about $1.32 per month per user or about 7¢ per day for a typical 21 day 'spontaneous remission'. No doctors, pharmaceuticals, shots, diets, medications, or other intervention appears necessary.

One compact battery-powered *blood* clearing instrument is basically a miniature relay driven by a timer chip set to ~4 Hertz. Its 0 to 27V user adjustable biphasic output minimizes electrode site irritation. The described system delivers stimulation through *normally circulating blood* via electrodes placed at selected sites (such as one electrode behind ankle bone on inside of foot and another on opposite foot) over the sural, popliteal, posterior tibial, or peroneal arteries where the subjects' blood vessels are accessibly close to the surface (pg. 7) or on wrist or arm. Optimum electrode positions are reliably located by feeling for strongest pulse (pg. 5.) Micro current, treatment is of such low amplitude that it creates no discomfort when used as directed and is demonstrated to have no harmful side effects on healthy blood cells or tissue. A major obstacle to this simple and obvious solution is contrived aversion and disbelief. Treating approximately 120 minutes per day for four or six weeks should in the writer's opinion effectively neutralize well over 95% of any HIV and simultaneously any other electrosensitive viruses, parasites, bacteria, or fungi in blood. In heavy infections, shorter application times could prevent overloading patients with toxins. Simply treat for a greater number of days or inject ozonized water. In time, the restored immune system plus silver colloid may handle residual problems. In the special case of diabetically impaired circulation longer treatment times may be indicated. (Refer to expanded instructions on pg. 5.) Immobilized viruses may be expelled naturally through kidneys and liver. More rapid neutralization is possible but *not* recommended because of potential excessive toxic elimination reactions (Herxheimer's syndrome). T-cell counts may drop initially because of lysing and subsequent scavenging by macrophages but should recover and increase after a few months. Even negative PCRs are sometimes reported.

Latent / germinating HIV reservoirs in the body's *lymph* or other tissue may theoretically be neutralized with a *second* and separate device by the strategy of generating a very high intensity (~10 kilogauss) short duration (~10 μS) magnetic pulse of ~20 joules by discharging a modified strobe light's capacitor through an applicator coil held at body points over lymph nodes, thymus, kidneys, adenoids, and other possible internal sites of latent infection (see pg. 8). By the physics of Eddy current / back emf "transformer action" (Lenz' law) the desired criteria of minimum current induced through infected tissue on the order of 100 μA to 1 mA should be readily attained. Several pulses repeated at each site may insure a reliable "overkill" for successful disease neutralization. A magnetic "pulser" is very inexpensive and simple to build. Full instructions are on pg. 6...

But subjects must assume responsibility for their own health - a "heresy" in today's society where we're conditioned to look for answers only to a medical establishment that has no current knowledge remotely promising "cures" for numerous other well known fatal diseases.

These "theoretical solutions" are being disclosed under constitutional freedom of speech guarantees in spite of extensively organized hostile opposition to non-pharmaceutical or *inexpensive* cures. Data can be *legally* offered only as "theoretical" and no medical claims can be made or implied. See your health professional! Anyone at his discretion and assumed responsibility should be free to build, use (on himself) and network his "research" results. With these data an average intelligent high school student should confidently be able to assemble *both* theoretical blood and tissue clearing modalities in about three hours and for a total investment of around $75.00. Components are widely available. After assembling, "cures" cost about $1.50 per patient for batteries. If electronically unskilled, 'busy' or technically illiterate, call an 'Amateur Radio Supply' store (yellow pages) and find a ham radio operator, hobbyist or TV repairman or pay any kid on the block to do it for you. After 'spontaneous remissions' some users may wish to interest their doctors. But be advised that *electronic* cures may be vigorously suppressed or ignored because there is presently no credibility nor drug cartel profit in this inexpensive AIDS solution. Also the 1910 Rockefeller/Flexner Report attempted to discredit Electro-medicine with a conspiracy to inflate pharmaceutical profits.

I'm definitely *not* soliciting funds. This was independently developed by Bob Beck at his private expense and offered freely for 'theoretical and informational purposes only' and with absolutely no profit motive. Non-FDA approved devices are illegal to use within the USA except via little known FDA regulation loopholes whereby doctors and *researchers* are allowed to use *anything* on patients if they build it themselves (Code of Federal Regulations 21 § 807.65 subsections (d) & (f)). See actual text in footnote on pg. 4. Although we will offer technical updates and always welcome feedback from users, please respect the writer's privacy and never attempt to contact him for additional help or construction information. *Everything* users need to know is included herein.

We have nothing for sale.

EXPERIMENTAL IN VIVO BLOOD VIRUS, MICROBE, FUNGI, AND PARASITE ELIMINATION DEVICE

Revision March 16, 1996 Copyright © 1993/1996 Robert C. Beck

Note: These data are for informational, Instructional, and research purposes only and are not to be construed as medical advice. Consult your licensed medical practitioner.

CHANGES since previous editions: Pulse Repetition Rate from 0.67 to ~4 Hz. (Not critical). C 2 from 1 to 0.22µF. Voltage from 36 to 27V. Treatment time increased to 2 hours daily for 21 to 30 days. Improved electrode design and single wrist electrode placement. SW 2 added to extend battery life. There are NO "errors" in this schematic. Hundreds have been constructed successfully when duplicated exactly without user attempted "improvements".

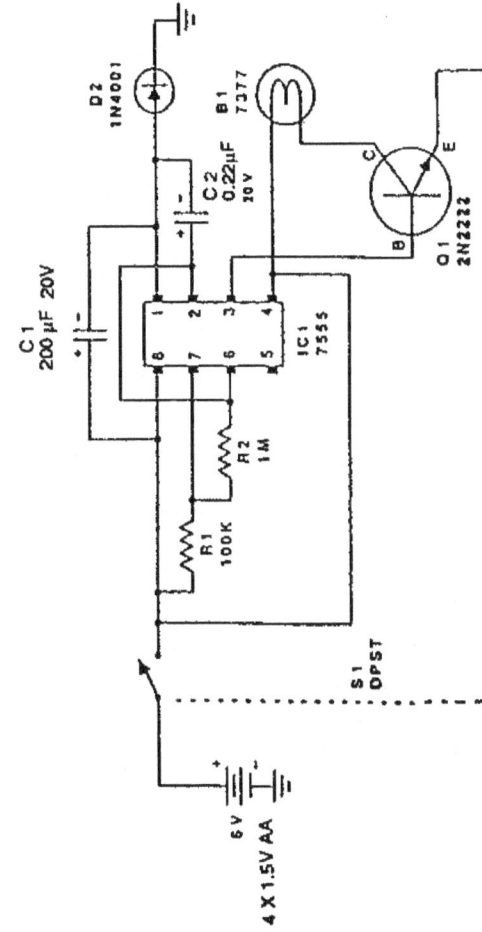

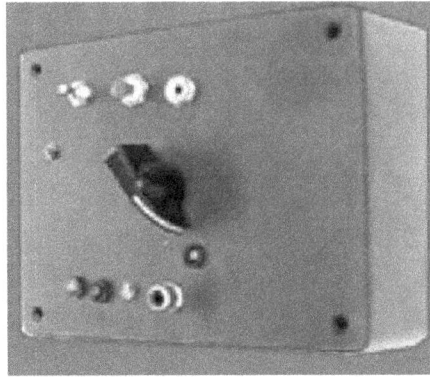

J1 (Electrodes)

R5
100K
Pot

SW2
"Test"
Momentary On

R3
2.2kΩ

D3
Zener
18V

D4
Zener
18V

LED 1

LED 2

DPDT
Relay

R4
1kΩ

D1
1N4001

27V
(3 X 9V)

B
E
C
2N2222
Bottom View

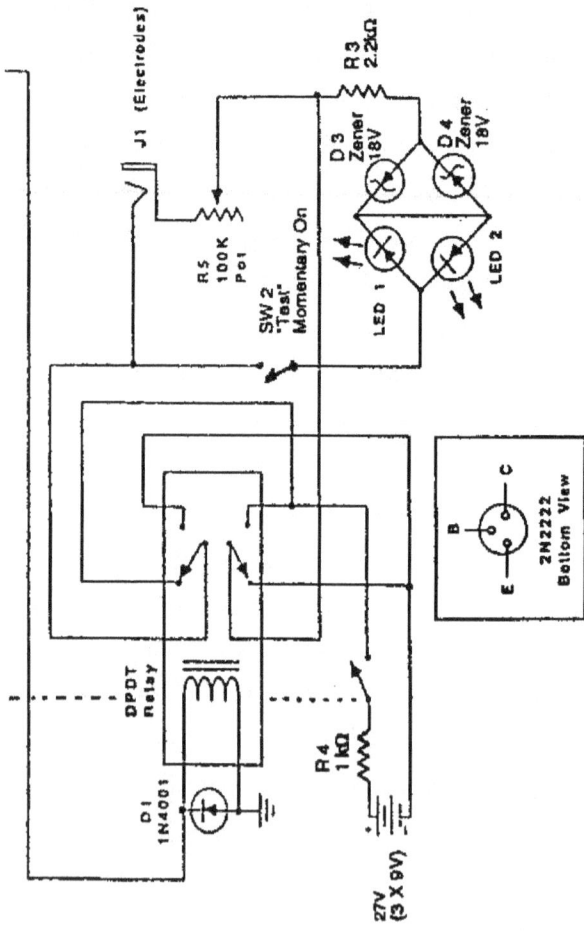

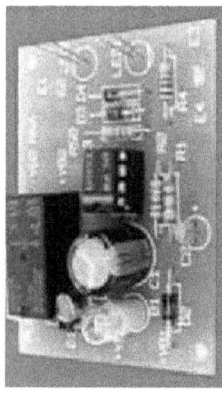

SPECIAL PARTS

B1: Filament type incandescent bulb, 6.3V .075A type 7377 (Ballast & current limiter.)
Relay: 5', 50 Ω coil, PCB mount DPDT; Selecta Switch SR15P207D1.
D3 & D4: Zener Diodes, 18V ½ watt NTE 5027A.
R5: 100kΩ ½ watt linear potentiometer; Caltronics P-68 or equiv.
LED I & 2, combined as Bicolor red & green in same housing, Radio Shack # 276-012
SW2: "Test" SPST momentary on subminiature push-button, Radio Shack # 275-1571

PROPOSED THEORETICAL IN-VIVO BLOOD HIV, PATHOGEN, PARASITE, NEUTRALIZING DEVICE

COMPONENT DESCRIPTIONS, SOURCES, AND CURRENT PRICES (March1995)
Revision March 13, 1996. Copyright © 1991/1996 Robert C. Beck

Note: These data are for theoretical, informational and instructional purposes only and are not to be construed as medical advice. Consult your licensed medical practioner. Note: Some builders have ego problems with following instructions *(Not Invented Here)* and like to find "mistakes" or possible "improvements". Hundreds have been built successfully if duplicated exactly as shown.

Do not expect this device to function optimally If ANY electrical changes or ego Improvements are attempted.

Component	Ref	Price
7555 CMOS timer chip (generic)	IC1	$1.80
100 k ohm ¼ watt 5% resistor	R 1	.07
1 meg Ω ¼ watt 5% resistor	R 2	.07
2.2k Ω ¼ watt 5% resistor	R 3	.07
1 k Ω ¼ watt 5% resistor	R 4	.07
100k Ω linear taper pot, ½ watt Caltronics P-68	R 5	2.56
200 µF 20 V (or higher) electrolytic capacitor	C 1	.45
0.22 µF 20 V (or higher) Tantalum capacitor	C 2	.25
1N4001 diode 2 required @ .15	D 1 & D 2	.30
18 Volt Zener diodes, ½ watt, 2 @ .79	D 3 & D 4	1.58 (NTE5027A)
NPN Transistor, generic 2N2222	Q1	.30
Bulb, 6.3 V .075 A type 7377	B1	1.34
Relay, 5 V 50Ω coil PCB Mount DPDT Selecta Switch	SR15P207D1	5.45
Misc. wire, solder, etc.		.50

Note: Action now supplies a custom printed circuit board #PS-PCB for: 15.00

They also have a complete kit available for about $80.00.

All 15 components listed above available at   ACTION ELECTRONICS
1300 E. Edinger, Santa Ana, CA 92705 (714) 547-5169

Bicolor LED red/green Radio Shack #276-012   LED 1 $ 1.19
Jack for electrode leads 274-251 #/$1.59   J 1   .53
DPDT switch, 275-626 or equiv. (Used as DPST)   SW 1   2.55
SPST Submini momentary push button switch   SW 2   .59   ER-SW101 "Test"
Battery Holder, 4-AA cells, Radio Shack 270-383   1.29
4 Alkaline AA cell batteries, #23-552 4 for   2.89
3 Alkaline 9V batteries, type 1604 etc. 3 for   3.75
3 9V battery snaps (clip-on connectors) #270-325 pkg 5/$1.29 1.29
Box, if used   2.29

Above items generally available at local Radio Shack Stores

Lead wire with 3.5 mm plug, 6 ft., Mouser or Calrad Electronics .35
Electrodes, stretch elastic, Velcro, cotton flannel, alligator clips, etc   ± 5.00   (See Notes)

Total Cost for all components for do-it-yourself project   **$ 49.24**

This design is basically a 7555 IC timer chip set for 50% duty cycle and ~3.9 Hz driving a subminiature relay. Electrode polarity continually reverses ~¼ second positive / ¼ second negative. Frequency is **not** critical.

Patents applied for.

Footnote:

CODE OF FEDERAL REGULATIONS 21 § 807.65 Subpart D - Exemptions, Paragraphs (d) & (f)
Excludes and exempts from regulation:

"(d) Licensed practitioners, including physicians, dentists, and optometrists, who manufacture or otherwise alter devices solely for use in their practice."

"(f) Persons who manufacture, prepare, propagate, compound, or process devices solely for use in research, teaching, or analysis, and do not introduce such devices into commercial distribution."

Use of this device therefore appears legal and exempt from FDA regulations when you construct it yourself for research and / or use in your own practice! But double-check your local, county and state regulations for possible exceptions.

This 11/24/'96 page describes a "Plant Growth Stimulator" improved since my 1991 design. User-tested for over two years, it is solid state (no relays), uses three (not seven) batteries, makes colloids, is much smaller, lighter, silent, with battery saving features, and is available as a mostly-assembled kit complete with electrodes and silver for about $100 from **Action Electronics**, 1300 E. Edinger Ave., Santa Ana, CA 92705 (714) 547 5169.

Colloids

RCA Jack

+27V

"Grain of Wheat"
Incandescent bulb
6-12V 55 mA
ML-612 or equiv

R8 150 Ω

**Biological
Electrification**

3.5 mm
Jack

R7 820 Ω

+27V

R5 100 kΩ linear
with SPST switch

C2 22 µF
25V.

CR 1

BiColor LED

D2

18V

B 1
9V

B 2
9V

D 1

18V

B 3
9V

(-)

R2 150 kΩ

U1A   **LM 358**

+27V

R1 2.4 meg Ω

U1B

C1 0.1 µF

R4 100 kΩ

R3 100 kΩ

+27V

OUTPUT: COLLOIDAL SILVER

OUTPUT: 4 Hz SQUARE WAVE

CIRCUIT DESCRIPTION

Copyright © 1996 Robert C Beck

The first section (U1A) of the LM 358 dual op-amp is a 50 volt peak-to-peak square wave oscillator. The second section (U1B) reverses polarity and provides ±27VDC output of low impedance. This delivers a biphasic, sharp rise-time output of ~4 Hz. (not critical) for the biological cotton-covered stainless-steel electrodes saturated with salt water before applying. Sharp rise-time is considered necessary to provide higher odd harmonics to the stimulus, although "rounded" waveforms will feel different.

The third section is a current-limited 27VDC output from a separate RCA jack for rapid generation of excellent colloidal silver in water. A three minute cycle in 8 Oz. of room-temperature water makes a ~3 ppm concentration.

Op-amp section 1A's 4 Hz oscillator frequency is set by C1 (0.1 μF) and R1 (2.4 megΩ). It is configured as a comparator with hysteresis determined by R2 (150 kΩ). Charging and discharging of C1 is done by the 180° out-of-phase signal through R1. R3 and R4 provide a set-point 1/2 the V+ to the comparator. This insures a 50% duty cycle square wave with an amplitude of slightly less than the ~27V supply.

U1B, the second comparator, is used to invert the output of oscillator U1A. A ~50V peak-to-peak signal will be generated between the op-amps due to their outputs being 180° out of phase. U1B's current is limited by potentiometer R5 (100 kΩ) and R7 (820 Ω) and is set to individual user's comfort.

The power indicator circuit consists of a bicolor (red-green) LED (CR1) and the series combination of two 18V Zener diodes, D1 & D2, with power limited by C2 (22 μF). This section of the device is automatically disabled when the 3.5 mm plug is inserted into it's jack. Therefore the LEDs flash only when batteries sum is over ~21V. If LEDs are dim or extinguished, replace with three fresh 9 V alkaline batteries. C2 used as a limiter allows the LED to flicker on at 1/8 intervals only as the square wave output reverses polarity.

Users find this newer design highly satisfactory, trouble free and most efficient.

EXPANDED INSTRUCTIONS FOR EXPERIMENTAL / THEORETICAL HIV BLOOD NEUTRALIZATION.
HYPOTHETICAL PROTOCOLS FOR EXPERIMENTAL SESSIONS

Revision March 20, 1997. Copyright © 1991/1997 Robert C. Beck

PRECAUTIONS: Do NOT use wrist to wrist with subjects with cardiac pacemakers. Any applied electrical signals may interfere with 'demand' type heart pacers and cause malfunction. Single wrist locations should be acceptable. Do NOT use on pregnant women, while driving or using hazardous machinery.

Users MUST avoid ingesting anything containing medicinal herbs, foreign or domestic, or potentially toxic medication. nicotine, alcohol, recreational drugs. laxatives, tonics. and certain vitamins etc., for one week before starting because blood electrification can cause electroporation which makes cell membranes pervious to small quantities of normally harmless-chemicals in plasma. The effect is the same as extreme overdosing which might be lethal. See *Electroporation: a General Phenomenon for Manipulating Cells and Tissues;* J.C. Weaver, Journal of Cellular Biochemistry 51:426-435 (1993). Effects can mimic increasing dosages many fold. Both the magnetic pulsar and blood purifier cause electroporation.

Do NOT place electrode pads over skin lesions, abrasions, new scars, cuts, eruptions, or sunburn. Do NOT advance output amplitude to uncomfortable levels. All subjects will vary. Do NOT fall asleep while using. The magnetic pulser should be safe to use anywhere on body or head.

Avoid ingesting alcohol 24 hours before using. Drink an 8 oz. glass of distilled water 15 minutes before and immediately following each session end drink at least four additional glasses daily for flushing during 'neutralization' and for one week thereafter. This is imperative. Ignoring this can cause systemic damage from unflushed toxic wastes. When absolutely essential drugs *must* be ingested, do so a few minutes *after* electrification then wait 24 hours before next session.

If subject feels sluggish, faint, dizzy, headachy, light-headed or giddy, nauseous. bloated or has flu-like symptoms or rashes after exposures, reduce pulsing per session and/or shorten applications of electrification. Drink more water- preferably ozonized - to speed waste oxidation and disposal. Use extreme caution when treating patients with impaired kidney or liver function. Start slowly at first like about 20 minuted per day to reduce de-toxification problems.

To avoid shock liability, use batteries only. Do NOT use any line-connected power supply, transformer, charger, battery eliminator, etc. with blood clearing device. However line supplies are OK with well-insulated magnetic pulse generators (strobe lights).

Health professionals - Avoid nicotine addicts, vegans, and other unconsciously motivated death-wishers and their covert agendas of 'defeat the healer'. Tobacco, the most addictive (4½ times more addictive than heroin) and deadly substance of abuse known, disrupts normal cardiovascular function. True vegetarian diets are missing essential amino acids absolutely necessary for the successful rebuilding of AIDS-ravaged tissues. Secondary gains (sympathy / martyrdom, work avoidance, free benefits, financial assistance, etc.) play large roles with many AIDS patients. "Recovery guilt" as friends are dying has even precipitated suicide attempts masked as 'accidents'. Avoid such entanglements, since many have unconscious death wishes.

SUPERIOR ELECTRODES. Excellent, convenient and vastly superior electrodes, reusable indefinitely can be made by butt-soldering lead wires to ends of 1⅛" long by 3/32" dia. blanks cut from type 316 stainless steel rods available from welding supply stores (Cameron Welding Supply, 11061 Dale Ave., Stanton, CA 90680). Use 'Sta y Clean' flux before soldering (zinc chloride/hydrochloric acid). Shrink-insulate TWO tight layers of tubing over solder joints to prevent flexing/breaking and lead/copper ions from migrating. Wrap three or four turns of 100% cotton flannel around rods. Spiral-wrap with strong thread starting from wire side to end, tightly pinch cloth over the rod's end so as to leave no metal exposed by wrapping 6 or 7 turns of thread TIGHTLY just off end of rod, then spiral wrap back to start and tie tightly with four knots then cut off excess cloth at end close to pinch-wraps. Treat end windings and knots with clear fingernail polish or Fray Check® (fabric & sewing supply stores) to prevent raveling. Soak in a strong solution of sea salt (not table salt) containing a little wetting agent like Kodak Photo Flow, ethylene glycol, or 409 kitchen cleaner. Add a few drops of household bleach, silver colloid, etc, for disinfectant. Store solution for reuse. Tape soaking wet electrodes tightly over pulse sites with paper masking or Transpore™ tape or with 1" wide stretch elastic bands with tabs of Velcro® at ends to fasten. Electrodes should closely conform precisely along blood vessels, not skewing ever so slightly over adjacent flesh. This insures better electrical conductivity paths to circulating blood and insures very low internal impedance (~2000Ω). Rinse and blot-dry electrodes and skin after each use. NEVER allow bare metal to touch skin as this will cause burns manifested as small red craters that heal slowly. The objective is to get maximum current into blood vessels, not leak it over to adjacent tissue. Therefore never use any electrode wider that about ⅛ inch.

ELECTRODE PLACEMENTS: Locate maximum pulse position (NOT to be confused with acupuncture, reflexology, Chapman, etc. points) on feet or wrists by feeling for maximum pulse on inside of ankle ~1" below and to rear of ankle bone, then test along top center of instep. Place electrode on whichever pulse site on that foot that feels strongest. Scrub skin over chosen sites with mild soap and water or alcohol swab. Wipe dry. Position the electrodes lengthwise along each left and right wrists blood vessel. Note: with subjects having perfectly healthy hearts and not wearing pacers, it is convenient to use left wrist to right wrist exactly over ulnar arterial pulse paths instead of on feet. Recent (Dec. 1995) research suggests that placing both electrodes over different arteries on the same wrist works very well (see pg. 7), avoids any current through heart, and is much more convenient and just as effective. An 8" long, 1" wide elastic stretch-band with two 1½" lengths of ¾" wide Velcro® sewn to ends of opposite sides makes an excellent wrist band for holding electrodes snugly in place. With electrode cable unplugged, turn switch ON and advance amplitude control to maximum. Push momentary SW. 2 'Test' switch and see that the red and green light emitting diodes flash alternately. This verifies that polarity is reversing ~4 times per second (frequency is NOT critical) and that batteries are still good. When LED's don't light replace all three 9V batteries. When the white incandescent bulb dims or appears yellowish, or relay isn't clicking, replace all four AA cells. Zener diodes will extinguish LEDs when the three 9V battery's initial 27V drops below 18V after extended use. Never use any electrode larger than 1⅛" long by ⅛" wide to avoid wasting current through surrounding tissue. Confine exactly over blood vessels only. Apply drops of salt water to each electrode's cotton cover ~every 20 minutes to combat evaporation and insure optimum current flow. Later devices are solid-state, use only three batteries and no relays, and are much smaller.

Now rotate amplitude control to minimum (counter-clockwise) and plug in electrode cable. Subject now advances dial slowly until he feels a "thumping" and tingling. Turn as high as tolerable but don't advance amplitude to where it is ever uncomfortable. Adjust voltage periodically as he adapts or acclimates to current level after several minutes. If subject perspires, skin resistance may decrease because of moisture, so setting to a lower voltage for comfort is indicated. Otherwise it is normal to feel progressively less sensation with time. You may notice little or no sensation at full amplitude immediately, but feeling will begin building up to maximum after several minutes at which time amplitude must be decreased. Typical adapted electrode-to-electrode impedance is on the order of 2000Ω. Typical comfortable input (to skin) is ~3mA, and maximum tolerable input (full amplitude) is ~7mA but this 'reserve' margin although harmless is unnecessary and can be uncomfortable. Current flowing through blood is very much lower than this external input because of series resistance through skin, tissue and blood vessel walls, but 50 to 100 µA through blood is essential.

Apply blood neutralizer for about 2 hours daily for ~2 months. Use judgment here. The limiting factor is detoxification. Carefully monitor subject's reactions (discomfort, catarrh, skin eruptions, weeping exudites, rashes, boils, carbuncles, coated tongue, etc.) With very heavy infections, go slower so as not to overload body's toxic disposal capability. With circulation-impaired diabetics, etc., you may wish to extend session times. Again, have subject drink lots of water. Recent changes in theoretical protocol being currently tested suggest following up the three weeks of treatments with a 24 hours per day (around the clock) continuous electrification of blood for two days to deal a knockout blow to the remaining HIV's 1.2 day life cycle. (A. Perelson, Los Alamos Biophysics Group, Mar. 16, 1996 'Science' Journal.) Remember to remoisten electrodes regularly. If you absolutely must ingest prescription drugs, do so immediately after turning off instrument and allow 24 hours before next treatment to let concentrations in blood plasma decay to lower levels.

Remember, if subjects ever feel sleepy, sluggish, listless, nauseous, faint, bloated, or headachy, or have flu-like reactions they may be neglecting sufficient water intake for flushing toxins. We interpret this as detoxification plus endorphin release due to electrification. Let them rest and stabilize for ~45 minutes before driving if indicated. If this detoxing becomes oppressive, treat every second day. Treating at least 21 times should 'fractionate' both juvenile and maturing HIV to overlap maximum neutralization sensitivity windows and interrupt 'budding' occurring during HIV cells' development cycles. Treatments are claimed to safely neutralize many other viruses, fungi, bacteria, parasites, and microbes in blood. See US patents # 5,091,152, 5,139,684, 5,188,738, 5,328,451 and others as well as numerous valid medical studies which are presently little known or suppressed. Also ingesting a few oz. of ~5 parts per million of silver colloid solution daily can give subjects a 'second intact immune system' and minimize or eliminate opportunistic infections during recovery phase. This miracle substance is pre-1938 technology, and unlike ozone is considered immune from FDA harassment. Silver colloid can easily be made at home electrolytically in minutes and in any desired quantities and parts per million strength for under 1¢ per gallon plus cost of water. It is ridiculous to purchase it for high prices. Colloid has no side effects, and is known to rapidly eliminate or prevent hundreds of diseases. Silver colloids won't produce drug resistant strains as will all other known antibiotics. No reasonable amount can overdose or injure users either topically, by ingestion, or medical professional injection. Refer to page 9 for complete instructions on successfully making your own.

SUGGESTIONS FOR ACQUIRING AND USING AN INDUCTIVELY COUPLED MAGNETIC PULSE GENERATOR FOR THEORETICAL LYMPH AND TISSUE HIV NEUTRALIZATION

Revision February 28, 1997. Copyright © 1991/1997 Robert C. Beck

Note: These data are for informational and instructional purposes only and are not to be construed as medical advice. Consult with your licensed health practitioner.

In keeping with do-it-yourself inexpensive hypothetical approaches to self-help, the simplest and most rapid means for obtaining a capacitor-discharge magnetic pulse **lymph and tissue pathogen neutralizer** would be to find and modify a used functioning portable battery *and* ac powered electronic flash (strobe light) for cameras. These are acquired at swap meets, yard sales, pawn shops, or in junk boxes at used camera stores. Or purchase a new Vivitar (brand) model 1900 ($22) carried at some professional camera stores. This compact, light weight, inexpensive, rapid recharging flash is only 17.5 Watt-seconds (Joules; calculated as ½ CV² where C is in μF and C is in kilovolts) power but is readily available and easily modified. It works well enough for casual use but runs on batteries only so has greater operating expense than an AC/DC unit.

California swap meet prices for *used* strobes range from $4.00 to about $18.00. One Sunday the writer found a dozen *ac/dc* strobes, all in good working condition. Carry four AA batteries with you so you can test flash units before purchasing. I chose to modify a long discontinued Vivitar (brand) model 110 because it was larger than the rest and seemingly more powerful, however almost any brand or model of comparable output power (35 watt-seconds) should work. *Preferably select one with 115V ac as well as battery operating (dc) capability.*

First wind the applicator coil. Junk VHS videocassette reels are cheap, plentiful and adequate for this application. Remove 5 screws from shell, remove reels and discard tape. Be SURE alternative spools (if used) are non-conductive or system will not work. Avoid shorter length VHS tape reels which may have center hubs larger than 1" dia. and won't hold sufficient wire. Drill ¼" holes through hub and through center of flange(s). Make two 4" discs from ¼" thick plastic or fiberboard, drill ¼" center holes and another ¼" hole off-center so coil's inside lead wire can be pulled through. These 'stiffeners' will sandwich reel's flanges so they won't warp or split as wire pressure builds up while winding progresses. A 2" (or longer) ¼-20 machine nut and bolt with washers through centers will clamp flange stiffeners and reel and also provide a shaft to hold in a variable speed drill motor or similar winding device if used. Then remove bolt and stiffeners.

Specifications: Completely fill tape spool with #14 or 16 enameled copper magnet wire (130 to 160 turns) wound onto the 1" dia. hub and 3-½" OD spool with a gap width for wire of ⅝". Scrape enamel insulation ½" from ends and tin. Pull inside end of magnet wire through hub and stiffener and to outside. ~130 turns (about About 1-½" ■ should fill spool. Remove bolt, stiffeners, and finished coil. Now solder ends of 3 ft of *heavy* two-wire extension cord to each side of coil. Finished coil weighs ~1 LB 3 oz, has ~0.935 millihenry inductance, 0.34 Ω resistance, and takes ~20 minutes to hand wind or ~3 minutes with drill motor. An excellent alternative is an AMS brand air-core crossover inductor for home audio. MCM Electronics, Centerville, OH 45459. (800) 543-4330 catalog # 50-940. #16 gauge, 0.58Ω, 2.5mH, 2-⅞" dia., $10.65

Strobe modification consists simply of wiring the finished applicator coil with 4' ft. leads in series between either flash tube electrode. Be extremely cautious when working with case open because a strobe's capacitor can hold a residual high-voltage charge for a long time even when 'off'. Before modifying and to avoid shock, short out the capacitor by placing clip leads directly across the flash tube. Remember to remove this shunt later. To install coil, unsolder either wire from flash tube and connect one lead wire from coil to the wire you just removed from tube. Insulate connections with tape. This places your coil *in series* with the flash tube and enables the tube to act as an ionized gas relay or 'thyratron' that dumps most of capacitor's stored energy through coil when fired. Lamp will still flash but less brightly. Cover flash window with black paper. Melt wire-slot with soldering iron. Replace case. You're done!

Is it working properly? A good way to test for strength of pulsed magnetic energy is to lay a thin *steel* washer (one strongly attracted to magnet) flat on top of coil, ½" off center. A 1" dia. 'fender' washer with ½" center hole works well. Let the flash unit charge for about ten seconds plus or until the strobe's 'ready light' comes on then push flash button and see how high the washer is 'kicked' by Eddy current repulsion. A 35 watt-second strobe repels a washer about 14 inches vertically. Think of your pulsed coil as the 'primary' of a transformer and anything conductive nearby (living tissue included) as the 'secondary' into which current is induced when cut by coil's time-varying magnetic lines of flux. Your do-it-yourself magnetic pulse generator delivers a measurable output intensity *several thousand times* more powerful during each cycle than $7,000.00 German "Magnetotrons"®, Elecsystem "Biotrons"®, or Canada's "Centurion"® devices widely exhibited at holistic medical expos, none of which is *nearly* powerful enough for HIV, herpes, hepatitis or Epstein-Barr neutralization or adequate electroporation. It is also functionally similar to the "Diapulse"® miracle-working healing modality when coil is applied over liver and other organs. Magnetic fields and therefore induced currents penetrate *all* body cells, bones and tissues in proximity to coil (effective approx. 4 inches deep) and can theoretically neutralize electro-sensitive pathogens and viruses such as herpes B, HIV, hepatitis, Epstein-Barr and possibly many others as yet undiscovered that can hide *within* nerve sheaths and are therefore untouchable via immune system, white cells, or injectables. This may account for the impossibility of curing many known chronic infections via pharmaceuticals, antibiotics, or any presently known conventional treatments other than electrotherapy. Use pulser on body sites daily before blood electrification. This pulser is safe to use anywhere on the head, and body except with cardiac pacemaker users. See pg. 8 for lymph gland locations. Zap sites at ~10 second intervals for ~ 20 minutes daily.

To use, press fully insulated coil flat against body over lymph glands and other selected locations such as shown on pg. 8. Let strobe build up to full charge (about 4 to 10 seconds between pulses) and fire coil while contacting each site. Subjects will feel no physical sensations except for light 'thumps' during this phase of treatment. Exposure levels are considered safe because intensity of this magnetic pulser is much lower than Magnetic Nuclear Resonance Imaging in routine use on tens of thousands of patients. But should subject feel 'headachy', nauseous, sluggish, or display flu-like symptoms after exposures with either of these two devices, reduce number of pulses or duration of blood clearing process and drink more water. If immune system is very badly damaged, you may need to repeat all routines after several months to insure permanent and complete neutralization. *When using, keep coil several feet away from credit cards, watches, magnetic tape, computers, floppy disks, homeopathic remedies, etc.,* since its powerful magnetic field can de-gauss and erase magnetic data as well as subtle energy potentized medicines. As an unanticipated serendipity, pulsers are reported to erase deeply rooted lymph and tissue pathology and possibly even classical "miasma's" as well as many other microbes, fungi, bacteria, parasites, and viruses. Flash should preferably be used with ac power to save battery costs since you'll only get about 40 full pulses per new set of alkaline batteries. For sanitary purposes, enclose coil in plastic zip-lock discardable sandwich. When treating numerous subjects if there's no ac adapter it is economical to utilize a small rechargeable lead-acid "motorcycle" battery. Sota Instruments, Vancouver Canada's latest pulser measures 600 μF, 330-350V; 36.75 Joules; 21,429 Gauss at 105 Amperes peak; 17,850 Ampere Turns; pulse rate time ~1.8 microseconds; pulse duration ~ 2.5 milliseconds; lifetime ~85,000 cycles; and penetrates ~8" through tissue.

How much should this cost? Used electronic flash lamps cost ~$2.00 to ~$18.00. Three ½ LB spools of #14 magnet wire retail for $9.66 ea. at Action Electronics. (You'll need ~1-½ LB) 4-AA alkaline batteries, $ 2.89. A 12 ft heavy duty #14 X 2-wire 15 amp. ac extension cord costs about $2.00 and makes 4 sets of leads, or use heavy-duty speaker wire. VHS spools ~50¢. Wholesale wire $2.50 to $4.35/ LB in 10 LB rolls at Pacific Wire & Cable, 1228 S. Village Way, Santa Ana, CA 92704. (714) 558-1864 ~1 week delivery. **~$12. minimum | $60.50 maximum.**

EASY LOCATION OF PREFERRED SITES FOR HYPOTHETICAL BLOOD ELECTRIFICATION

Revision January 10, 1997. Copyright © 1997 Robert C. Beck, D.Sc.

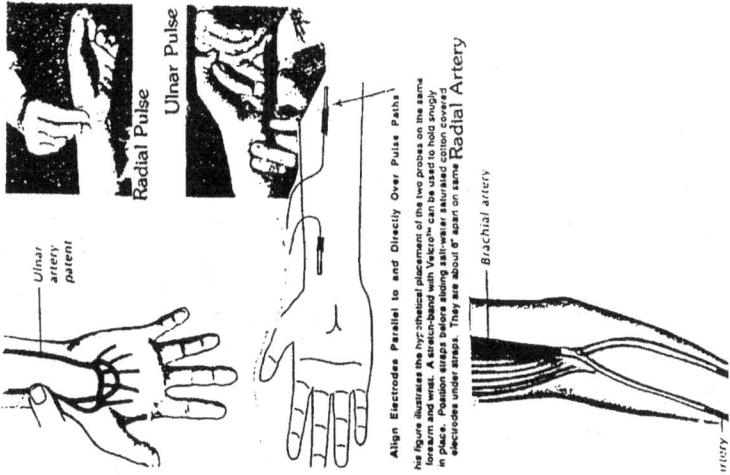

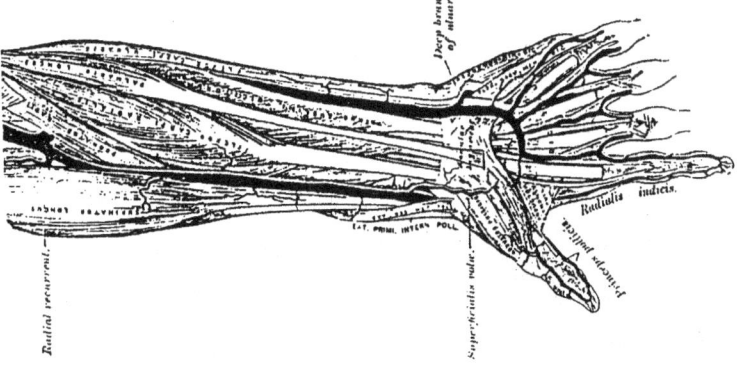

FIG. 504.—The radial and ulnar arteries.

FIG. 505.—Ulnar and radial arteries. Deep view

Radial Pulse

Ulnar Pulse

Align Electrodes Parallel to and Directly Over Pulse Paths

This figure illustrates the hypothetical placement of the two probes on the same forearm and wrist. A stretch-band with Velcro™ can be used to hold snugly in place. Position straps before sliding salt-water saturated cotton covered electrodes under straps. They are about 6" apart on same Radial Artery

Ulnar artery patent

Brachial artery

...artery

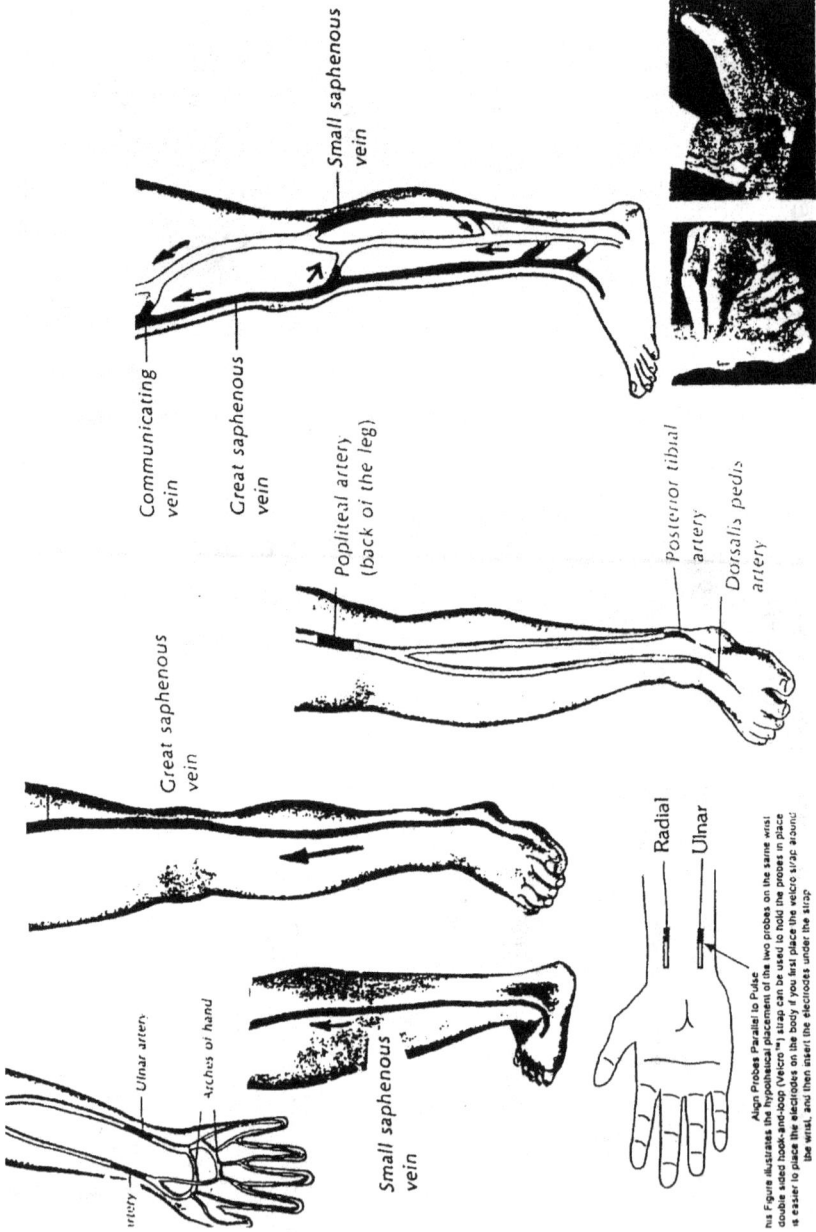

Small saphenous vein

Communicating vein

Great saphenous vein

Popliteal artery (back of the leg)

Posterior tibial artery

Dorsalis pedis artery

Great saphenous vein

Ulnar artery

Arches of hand

artery

Small saphenous vein

Radial

Ulnar

Align Probes Parallel to Pulse

This Figure illustrates the hypothetical placement of the two probes on the same wrist. A double sided hook-and-loop (Velcro™) strap can be used to hold the probes in place It is easier to place the electrodes on the body if you first place the velcro strap around the wrist, and then insert the electrodes under the strap

EASY LOCATION OF LYMPH NODES FOR PREFERRED HYPOTHETICAL
MAGNETIC PULSING SITES

JAN. 10, 1997 Revision. Copyright © 1997 Robert C. Beck, D.Sc.

Press either flat side of coil tightly into skin and "flash" each site three to five pulses daily _after_ "ready" lamp lights.

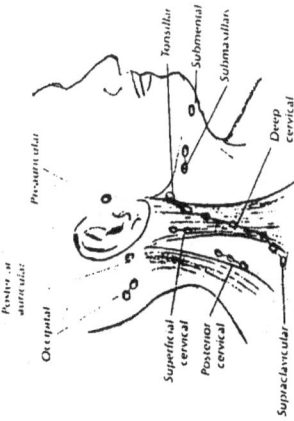

Right lymphatic duct.

Intercostal glands.

Lumbar

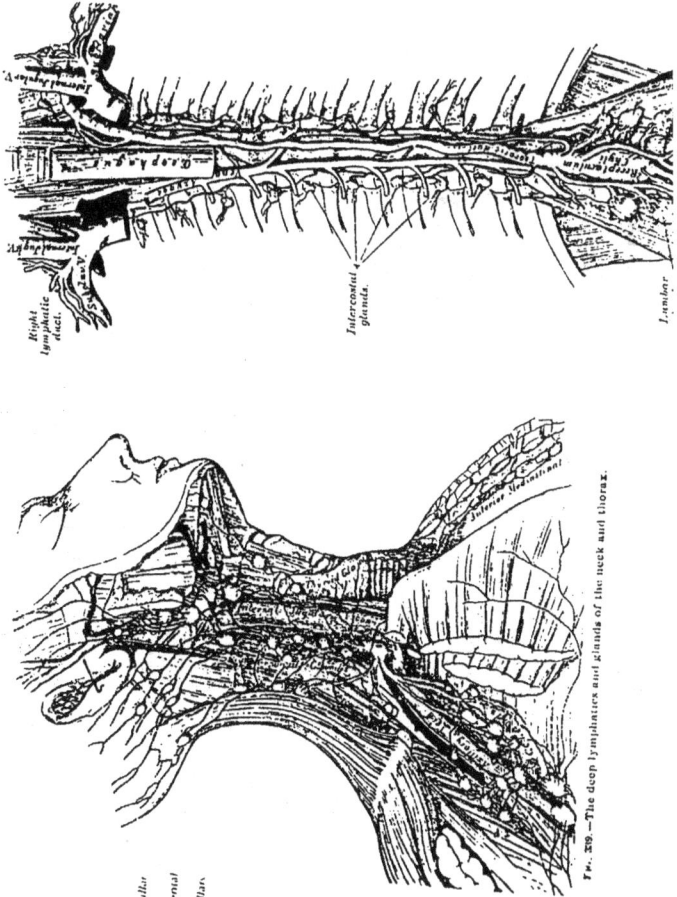

Inferior Mediastinal.

Fig. 339.—The deep lymphatics and glands of the neck and thorax.

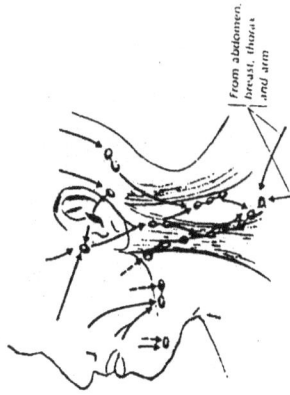

Posterior auricular

Occipital

Preauricular

Tonsilar

Submental

Submaxillary

Deep cervical chain

Superficial cervical

Posterior cervical

Supraclavicular

LYMPH NODES OF THE HEAD AND NECK

From abdomen, breast, thorax and arm

from mouth and throat

— External lymphatic drainage.
--- Internal lymphatic drainage.

LYMPHATIC DRAINAGE OF THE HEAD AND NECK

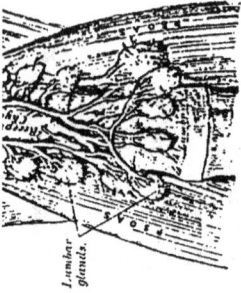

Lumbar glands.

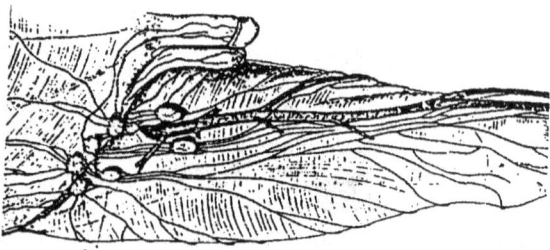

Fig. 317.—The thoracic and right lymphatic duct.

Superficial inguinal glands.

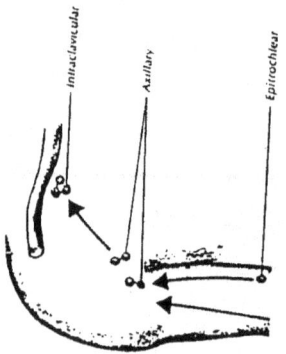

Intraclavicular

Axillary

Epitrochlear

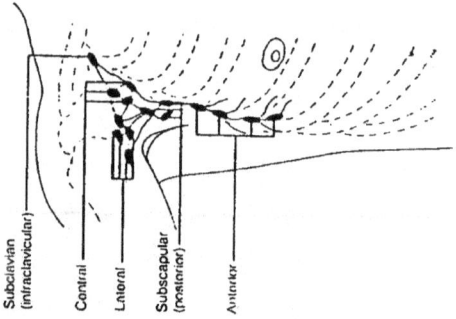

Subclavian (intraclavicular)

Central

Lateral

Subscapular (posterior)

Antorior

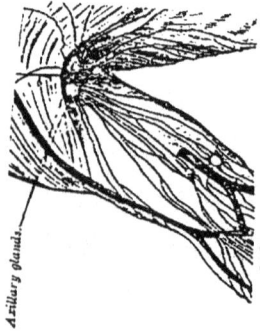

Axillary glands.

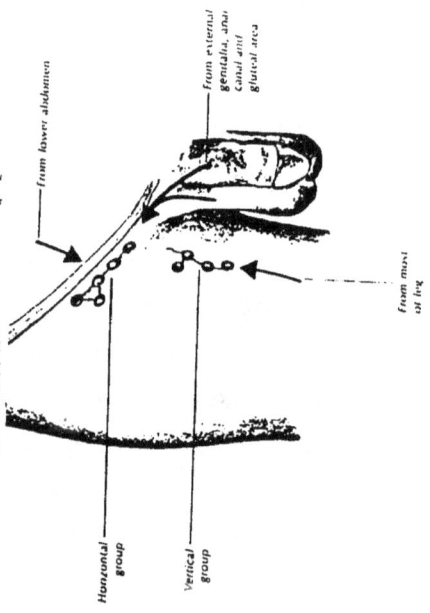

from lower abdomen

from external genitalia, anus canal and gluteal area

from most of leg

Horizontal group

Vertical group

Total Cancer Remissions through Blood Electrification Combined with Magnetic Pulsing plus Silver Colloid Ingestion

Theories Offered for Information and Educational Purposes Only and are the Author's Opinions

My archives contain a tantalizing report from several decades ago describing an authenticated record of an older man who was struck by lightning, survived, and subsequently grew a third set of teeth and a bushy head of youthful new dark hair. His grossly metastasized, inoperable cancers vanished. He threw away his glasses and cane, and appeared much younger and was totally healthy for the first time ever. This fascinated scientists and years later almost encouraged some highly illegal and bizarre human experiments in an abandoned aircraft hangar in Wendover, Utah where Tesla coil research with ball lightning was underway. The incident generated wide speculation but few insights at the time. This mystery remained sleeping until 1990 when an astounding discovery was reported at Albert Einstein College of Medicine in NYC by Drs. Kaali and Wyman. Not surprisingly, these data were apparently immediately suppressed. (See *Science News*; Mar. 30, '91 pg. 207; and *Longevity:* Dec.' 92 pg. 14.)

As a totally unexpected and unpredictable outcome of my self-funded research since 1991 into "blood electrification" with micro currents for AIDS (currently showing excellent results) a growing number of users previously unknown to me, began independently reporting remarkable "spontaneous remissions" of numerous *other* diseases *Including cancer.* Most involved no doctors, medication, or time off. Recoveries occurred after subjects had self-administered an altered do-it-yourself in vivo blood electrification treatment patially described as an In Vitro process in US Patent #5,188,738 issued to Dr. Steven Kaali in '93. (This work may have been anticipated twenty years earlier in 1973 by patent # 3,753,886 and by several others dating back to the turn of the century....) We were puzzled to find explanations. This preliminary report offers one possible theory. The magnetic pulser success with Cancer was independently proven in 1984 and described in US Patent #4,665,898 and eleven other independent researchers and patents going back over fifty years.

The Einstein disclosure describes removing blood from one arm, electrifying it, and returning it to the other arm in a process similar to dialysis. It also describes surgically implanted active electrode chambers containing miniature batteries sewn inside blood vessels. This author's preferred approach leaves all blood in the body, is totally non-invasive, costs practically nothing and is safely accomplished in about a month with ~two hours per day exposures as one goes about his normal activities. It handles most pathogens while blood flows naturally through the ~60cc volume of the electrified forearm's ulnar branch arteries from elbow to wrist. Without medications, invasive techniques or doctors, most pathogens, viruses, microbes, parasites and fungi just tend to disappear. Progress can be easily observed with dark-field and phase-contrast microscopy. The entire process and simple apparatus is fully described in my '91 paper and recent issues of **Explore**. (Vol. 7 #1.) Also simple instructions for self-made silver colloids of far better quality than you can usually buy are given. You can turn any glass of tap or distilled water into a 3 ppm top quality colloid in about two minutes anywhere with a shirt pocket battery-operated instrument. To date many "spontaneous remissions" of dozens of "incurable" illnesses including HIV have been reported by users and researchers of this "blood purification" when combined with ingestion of pennies-per-gallon instantly self-made silver colloid. Since none of dozens of friends using these apparent miracles has experienced infections, colds, flu, pneumonia, or lost a single day's productivity in over three years, evidence strongly suggests restored immune systems or dramatically improved blood functioning. It is also fascinating to note that several pet owners report their cats now refuse to drink water if silver colloid is not added. Trips to veterinarians with previously recurring infections were cut dramatically. It is as though the Creator had left a secret "back door" method for mankind to finally conquer incurable diseases plaguing us since the beginning of time. To stay out of big trouble, these data are being offered under "First Amendment freedom of speech" rights and legally should not be construed as medical advice.

It has long been known that dissections of cadavers dying of natural causes reveal many have had cancer several times during their lifetime resulting in "spontaneous remissions" generally without their knowledge and without ever visiting a doctor. An optimally functioning immune system somehow "handles" diseases of which the subject seldom becomes aware. Several promising broad-spectrum natural immunological agents like interferon and interleukin are produced by healthy Immune systems but would cost thousands for patients with already overloaded or "shut down" defenses although many such neuropeptides could speed cures. Other respected researchers describe "pleomorphic" forms of cancer pathogens which evolve through several stages- even mycotoxin involvement- *all* of which surrender to blood cleaning. In spite of dozens of theories offered, most diseases disappear with these simple, rapid, inexpensive in-vivo do-it-yourself tools and *without* drugs, herbs, homeopathics, pharmaceuticals, diets, doctors, discomfort or *any* medical intervention. Users have nothing to buy except replacement batteries. Complete recoveries cost under $2 per patient per disease. For persons unable to self-assemble the simple electrifier (about two hours and ~$30), dozens of people are currently custom building them and several companies are providing excellent and reliable combination "plant growth stimulators" and colloid generators ready to use. Most retail from $125 to $200. But this health breakthrough is politically incorrect and may never be FDA approved because of billions invested in treatment facilities, pharmaceuticals, and in clinical diagnostic equipment which must be amortized even if made obsolete. This discovery gives power over diseases back to the individual; an economic disaster for the health cartels. The only dangers lie in too rapid detoxification avoidable by increasing water intake for flushing wastes (Herxheimer's syndrome), plus ingestion of any herbs (even garlic) during blood electrification because of vastly enhanced cell absorption due to electroporation. (See J.C. Weaver; Harvard-MIT in *Journal of Cellular Biochemistry* 51:426-435; 1993.) All drugs, herbs, alcohol, tobacco, and some vitamins *must* be discontinued for at least two days before starting and for the duration of blood electrification or magnetic pulsing. This minimizes substances in your blood plasma which can become toxic at ~20X their normal levels.

Electrification is now being successfully used underground around the world. One Eastern MD claims numerous documented cancer cures by using only blood electrification and *no* surgery, radiation, drugs or chemotherapy. Many were considered terminal. We're even seeing clean blood tests of now healthy patients with previously long-standing Lupus. We have in our posession many IRB's showing complete HIV remissions, sero-conversions, and negative PCR tests.

The most reasonable theory of why electrification is so surprisingly effective for so many conditions lies in the now-proven fact that when correctly applied directly into blood (*not* into other body tissue like palms of hands, soles of feet, or organs) it neutralizes all microbes, pathogens, fungi, parasites, viruses, bacteria, mycotoxins and coexisting foreign lifeforms and alien invaders and their byproducts. This should never be confused with Royal Rife or Hulda Clark technology. Effective results are found to require a *minimum* of 27 Volts under load with low impedance output which must deliver up to several *milli*amperes measurable current into skin to produce the required 50 to 100 *micro*amperes internally through blood after the inevitable series resistance losses through vessel walls plus several layers of tissue. Electrical currents in blood can be measured with an ac microamp meter by IR drop using partially insulated hypodermic needles inserted ~6 inches apart into the same artery. Clark's "syncro zap" running at her standard 30 khz (considered many octaves too high to be effective) actually measures only ~2.6V peak to peak under load (~2000 ohms) at palms. This is an order of magnitude too low to have any real effect beyond placebo. The syncro-zapper's current is unmeasurable directly in the blood and physically cannot produce the essential 50 to 100 µA required internally. This may only mask readouts of parasite presence radionically. Unfortunately the live bugs remain undisturbed and are still there and will still be observed in stool and microscopic blood diagnosis. To function at all, electrification requires cotton-covered salt water saturated stainless steel electrodes *never* over 3/32" wide and 1" long. These must be carefully positioned directly over and precisely in line with arterial pulse points on opposite sides of the same wrist. This maximizes current into blood by not wasting it in surrounding tissue. Square or round TENS, EKG, EEG, EMG, etc. electrodes work only marginally and should never be substituted. Preferred instrument pulse-repetition rate is ~4 Hz biphasic with steep rise time and 50% duty cycle. Rate is *not* critical although much higher frequencies and certainly higher harmonics of the essential square wave output are degraded by "skin effect" where currents travel around the outside of body instead of internally. This is demonstrated by lighting a bulb in one hand while touching a Tesla coil with the other and not getting shocked. Electrification causes no known harmful side effects to healthy cells or tissue. A restored and unencumbered immune system may make one almost immortal I Electrified blood cells are observed to live for well over a month when sealed under cover slips on microscope slides while the average life of "normal blood is ~4 days. This strongly suggests that even aging bodies may easily and rapidly be made impervious to many hostile, toxic, infectious, antibiotic-resistant and even yet undiscovered invaders. The subject is barely scratched with miracles being reported regularly ranging from dramatic weight loss to restored hair, feature symmetry (Prof. R. Thornhill, Univ. N. Mexico), etc., many of which were totally unexpected but that I have personally experienced or observed.

One example- cervical cancer alone kills ~⅓ of all victims in the third world, and has long been known to be caused by the papilloma virus. Electrification eliminates these toxic "fellow travelers" coexisting in our blood and automatically handles innumerable diseases previously considered "incurable". Ebola or other possibly genetically engineered biological warfare "designer" germs may be unleashed someday per some theories of Gulf War Syndrome diseases which are currently immune to all other known countermeasures *except* blood electrification and colloids.

Like all revolutionary ideas, this incredible breakthrough barely survived initial ridicule and rejection because it is too startling, effective, inexpensive, simple and foolproof to be believable. It has experienced violent opposition from entrepreneurs selling health products made obsolete. Next, massive resistance came from the population's ~85% harboring unconscious hidden agendas or "death wishes" of "defeat the healer" and who must protect their secondary gains. And almost universally, people simply refuse to take responsibility for their own health. They think the "Doctor" priesthood should know what's "best" for them. And predictably, some doctors realize this will erode their incomes because it is cheap, universally effective, simple "do it yourself at home", and cures many things they can't. (A patient *cured* is a customer lost!) So acceptance of blood electrification is just now emerging to enthusiastic acceptance from those who've experienced the results. Being profit-motivated, the establishment must resist anything like this. But we now have our "hundredth monkey". Skeptics have only to use this technology to directly enjoy immensely better health. ***Take back your power! This works!***

The writer is a researcher, not a practitioner. **I have nothing for sale.** Please never try to contact me by phone or letter or through third parties since it is a felony for me to answer well meaning medical questions. I am a physicist, not a licensed medical practitioner and such devices are not presently FDA approved. But I am preparing a do-it-yourself photo illustrated manual covering all details which should be available by the end of this year.

Currently Preferred Silver Colloid Making Apparatus, Means, and Methods

To easily and rapidly make unlimited quantities of good quality silver colloid concentrate for ~1/10¢ per gallon plus water costs you'll need three 9V type MN1604 regular alkaline transistor radio batteries, three battery snap-on lead connectors, 2 insulated alligator clips, 1 "grain-off-wheat" 24 volt 40 mA sub miniature incandescent bulb, a foot of 3/32" heat-shrink insulation tubing, 10" pure silver wire, and a foot of 2-conductor stranded insulated wire for clip-leads. This should cost under $20 maximum for everything and take about 35 minutes to assemble from scratch. This design is "idiot proof" and simple to use. It makes an odorless, tasteless, colorless fast and powerful antiseptic and one of the most remarkable healing agents known. The entire colloid making process takes about five minutes per 8 OZ batch for ~5 ppm laboratory tested concentration at room temperature.

Use three snap-on connector clips for the batteries. Solder them in series (red to black) to provide 27 volts. Connect a 24V incandescent lamp in series with either (positive or negative) output lead. Solder a red insulated alligator clip to the positive (anode) and a black insulated dip to the negative (cathode) 2-conductor lead wires. Insulation is shrunk over soldered connections using a heat gun or match. Use ONLY pure silver (.999 fine) electrodes. #14 gauge (AWG) is the preferred size. Pure silver is sometimes available at electroplating supply companies, foundries, precious metals dealers, etc. Do NOT use "Sterling" silver (.9275 or other) since Sterling contains cooper and nickel. Nickel can be toxic. *WARNING!* Sterling is sometimes passed off for electrodes with commercial colloid makers through ignorance or by entrepreneurs who are trying to cut corners and save money. Discard them as hazardous. Use only triple distilled or de-ionized water for injectable colloid. Single distilled water makes transparent colloids but its higher resistance takes up to half an hour to make a 5 ppm. concentration. Tap water is O.K. for most other uses but contains chlorine which may produce some AgCl which is harmless but gives a milky appearance as will any salt (NaCl) which should be avoided.

Bend top ends of silver electrode wires to dip over rim of plastic or glass container. Leave about 4 inches of bare electrodes submergible in the working solution (water). Spacing between electrodes is not critical. There is no on-off switch, so process starts immediately when alligator dips are both attached to submerged wires. Process stops when either or both dips are disconnected. If bulb glows visibly, proceed and let current flow for about five minutes then remove alligator clips, stir, and you're done! If bulb doesn't light or you see only a faint reddish glow, add sea-salt solution (see next paragraph). Observe the smoke-like plumes of pure white ultra fine grain silver against a dark background as colloid electrolytically sinters off the anode (positive polarity side of battery; red lead) and drifts into solution. Stir thoroughly before using or storing and shake each time before using. Five minutes activation of ~8 OZ of properly conductive water at ~72F gives ~5 ppm (parts per million) strength. Ech additional 10° F will double ppm for a given electrolysis time. Yield also depends on water conductivity, surface area of electrodes, amount of current, and time. ~5 minutes makes a stock solution which can be safely used full strength for anything. I occasionally put electrodes in my coffee, fruit and vegetable juice, tap water, and other restaurant drinks to charge them with colloid directly. I even treated a mug of Anchor Steam Beer to see if it worked - it did! But its best to charge water by itself and add this to other foods and liquids as desired or drink it directly. Overdosing with any amount is considered unlikely.

The 24v, 40 mA miniature bulb acts as an ideal ballast, current limiter, and battery condition check for the apparatus. I found aircraft "grain-of-wheat" lamps (Precision Lamp, Inc. part #1028) in surplus for 50¢ each. You can momentarily short-circuit clip-leads together without harm; the bulb will simply light brightly. Also the visual brightness while operating gives an accurate indication of water conductivity. With distilled or de-ionized (high resistance) water, you should stir in a very minute amount (1 drop, no more) of dissolved sea salt solution, preferably "Celtic Golden Marine" (brand) available at health food stores. Do not use table salt since it contains additives like iodine, aluminum, or silica desiccates, etc. Too much salt (more then one drop) NaCl, can produce unwanted silver chloride and give a "dish water" appearance. Prepare a saturated solution of sea salt beforehand, filter and store in a 1 or 2 OZ brown drugstore eyedropper bottle. Add a little colloid to your bottle to prevent bacterial growth. Stir a drop of this salt solution into 8 Oz of any high-resistance water. The bulb should show just a very dim reddish glow. Salt must be added before making colloid. Make and store only in electrically non-conductive containers such as dark brown glass or plastic such as prune juice bottles, hydrogen peroxide containers, Kahlua or Bailey's Irish Cream liquor containers etc., but never in metal (don't peel labels as these shut out more light). Suggested adult dosage of silver colloid can be one to several OZ. stock solution in 6 to 8 OZ of water taken not more than three times in 24 hours. Consult your health professional. 8 OZ glasses of full strength (up to 30 p.p.m.) can be ingested directly with no harmful side effects.

Clean electrode wires after each use to remove dark oxide occurring on anode because the oxygen (produced electrolytically) oxidizes silver. Cut a small piece of ¼" thick nylon Scotchbright™ kitchen scouring pad to polish dried silver, then wipe with paper napkin to make silver ready for next use. A fresh set of 3 alkaline batteries will make hundreds of 8 Oz batches of five minute silver colloid before battery replacement becomes necessary. Periodically check batteries by momentarily short-circuiting tips of alligator clips together to observe whiteness and intensity of light. When bulb appears significantly dimmer or locks yellowish after time, replace all three alkaline batteries. Pry snap connectors off, tape 3 new cells together, and replace snap-on clips. Be very careful not to crush or damage the fragile little in-series lamp.

Colloid concentration and purity is readily checked by viewing back-scatter of a laser beam as it passes through your finished solution Tyndall/Rayleigh effect). Use a 1 to 5 milliwatt laser diode pointer (630 to 670 nanometer wavelength) that makes a small spot at several feet, not just a "light emitting diode". Look into the beam at about a 15 degree angle. (Point beam through solution so spot hits your chin or lips. Never look directly at source; this can injure your eyes.) Laser pointers retail for about $30. at some computer or parts outlets such as Fry's Electronics. Surprisingly the inexpensive pointer from Radio Shack does not perform satisfactorily for this particular application. Other Radio Shack models (~$69) will.

Stir your fresh batch with a plastic (non-conductive) fast-food disposable knife and store in a dark brown container. Keep away from light as even room light levels will degrade colloids rapidly by turning solution gray or black just as exposure to light darkens the silver in camera film. Light can also neutralize positive charges on silver ions that help keep particles in suspension. Keep colloids cool but do not refrigerate or let freeze. Always shake container thoroughly before using. After evaluating many different instruments and methods, this paper describes what is easily the best performing, least expensive. simplest and most convenient method for producing good quality silver colloids presently disclosed. It has been fully tested and found to work much better than expensive, dangerous and complex devices. However it does not work with metals such as gold. This standalone appliance works all by itself and never requires high voltage, ignition coils, transformers, underwater sparking, or "plugging in". It goes in your pocket and will work anywhere. It is essential for sterilizing local drinking water when traveling. (See accompanying suggested uses). It can generate excellent fine-grain silver colloids directly in any fluid containing water ranging from soup to champagne without diluting it. You can make any desired concentration in parts per million by electrolyzing at higher temperatures. There is no heat or waste, and it cannot shock you. There is no need to stir during processing however stirring or shaking is essential before storing and each time before using. Filtering is generally unnecessary. Don't add preservatives, minerals, EDTA, proteins, gelatin. coloring (some makers add yellow dye to make it appear "golden" and even honey to slow precipitation), or any other substances. If purchased at market prices commercial colloids could cost up to $60 for 8 OZ of generally vastly inferior products. Most available colloids on today's market when evaluated prove to be practically worthless. (At a recent health expo, in my opinion out of eight brands tested only two were found to be adequate in quality, suspension, and content. Many contained additives such as EDTA, coloring and gelatin for suspension). This paper describes an easy way for anyone to make his own for only a small fraction of a penny. It seems ridiculous to buy it for high prices. You can now afford to use colloids universally, such as in laundry water for sterilization, as a disinfectant spray, rinse for fruit and vegetables, fungicide, bactericide, plant spray, pet health assurance, and hundreds of other applications. Drinking dilute silver colloid safely kills over 650 pathogens, viruses. microbes. fungi, and parasites within minutes and is said to give you a second intact immune system. Side effects or overdosing are unknown and resistant strains of disease-causing pathogens never develop. Some users ingest lactobacillus acidophilus. bulgaricus, yogurt etc. to replenish friendly intestinal flora.

Warning! Multi-level entrepreneurs hoodwinked by profit motivated promoters generally protest that their colloid is "better, finer-particle size, purer, improved suspension, more golden, made by some expensive top secret proprietary process. etc." or other absurd rationalizations to justify outrageous prices. Just offer to test both at an independent laboratory. This do-it-yourself process makes a perfectly satisfactory colloid with a four year track record of excellent results. Should you wish to make "golden yellow" silver colloid, simply start with 8 Oz of distilled water, add no salt or soda or other ionizing material, and leave electrodes in for 30

A FEW UNIQUE PLUS TRADITIONAL USES FOR SILVER COLLOID

When you control a source of penny-per-gallon make-it-yourself high concentration silver colloid (see attached how-to page) you can use it for hundreds of health improvement applications. A few are suggested here. You can use most tap water to make colloid for industrial and external uses and distilled or de-ionized water for internal or injectable applications.

Add to suspected drinking water when traveling or camping. Colloid sprayed burns heal rapidly without scarring. Safely sterilize anything from toothbrushes to surgical instruments. Use topically on cuts, wounds, abrasions, rashes, sunburn. razor nicks, bandages. Spray on garbage to prevent decay odors. Mist kitchen sponges, towels, cutting boards to eliminate E. Coli 0157:H7 and salmonella bacteria to prevent food poisoning, gastrointestinal inflammation, and genital tract infections.

Add when canning, preserving, bottling. Use like peroxide on zits and acne. Add to juices and milk. Will delay spoiling, fermenting, deteriorating, clabbering or curdling. Spray in shoes, between toes, between legs to stop most skin itch, athletes foot, fungi, jock itch. Diminish dandruff, psoriasis, skin rashes, etc. Add to bath water, gargle, douches, colon irrigation, nasal spray and dental water-pic solutions. Cuts downtime dramatically with colds, flu, pneumonia, staph, strep, respiratory infections and rhino viruses. Skin itch, eye and ear infections, some moles and warts vanish when colloid is sprayed on body after bathing. Use with Q-tip on fingernail, toenail, and ear fungi. Neutralize tooth decay and bad breath. Colloid stops halitosis by eliminating bacteria deep in throat and on back of tongue. Unlike pharmaceutical antibiotics, silver colloid never permits strain-resistant pathogens to evolve.

Put a few drops on band-aids and bandages to shorten healing times. Health professionals might consider IV and IM injections. Tumor and polyp shrinking is reported when masses are injected directly (when colloid is added to sterile physiological saline or Ringer's Solution which contains ~9000 ppm sodium chloride). Toothaches, mouth sores, bacterial irritations are diminished. Soak dentures. Spray refrigerator, freezer and food storage bin interiors. Stop mildew and wood rot. Mix in postage stamp, envelope, and tape moistening wells, paint and paste pots to prevent bacterial growth, odors, spoiling or souring. Add to water based paints, wallpaper paste, dishwater, cleaning and mopping solutions, etc. Spray pet bedding and let dry.

Spray on top of contents of opened jam, jelly, and condiment containers and inside lids before replacing. Mix a little in pet water, birdbaths, cut flower vases. Always add to swamp cooler water. Spray air conditioner filters after cleaning. Swab air ducts and vents to prevent breeding sites for germs. Use routinely in laundry final rinse water and always before packing away seasonal clothes. Damp clothes or towels and washcloths will not sour or mildew. Eliminate unwanted microorganisms in planter soils and hydroponics systems. Spray plant foliage to stop fungi, molds, rot, and most plant diseases.

Treat pools, fountains, humidifiers, Jacuzzis, hot tubs, baths, dishwashers, recirculating cooling tower water, gymnasium foot dips, and bath and shower mats. Spray inside shoes, watch bands and gloves and under fingernails periodically. Treat shower stalls, tubs, fonts, animal watering troughs, shavers to avoid trading germs. Rinse fruit and vegetables before storing or using. Put in cooking water. Human and animal shampoos become disinfectants. Prevent carpets, drapes, wallpaper from mildewing. Wipe telephone mouthpieces, pipe stems, headphones, hearing aids, eyeglass frames, hairbrushes, combs, loofas. Excellent for diapers and diaper rash.

Do toilet seats, bowls, tile floors, sinks, urinals, doorknobs. Kill persistent odors. Rinse invalid's pillowcases, sheets, towels and bedclothes.

There are literally thousands of other essential uses for this ridiculously inexpensive, odorless, tasteless, colorless, totally benign and easily produced powerful non-toxic disinfectant and healing agent. You'll find that a spray or misting bottle of silver colloid solution may be the most useful health enhancement tool in your environment.

QUICK SUMMARY

A New Paradigm for Instant Healing

Disclosed here is a revolutionary do-it-yourself, safe, natural, inexpensive _proven_ solution to infectious diseases based on blood electrification. It requires no doctors, drugs, or other outside intervention. It costs practically nothing. Clinical tests have confirmed these four steps can "cure" HIV (AIDS), CANCER, HEPATITIS, LUPUS, EPSTEIN-BARR, GULF WAR SYNDROME, GIARDIA, CANDIDA, and even the common cold, plus most other known infectious diseases including ones for which there are no currently successful antibiotics, vaccines, or treatments. It is offered to humanity as a no-profit, information-only, empowerment for everyone who wishes to be healthy again. We have nothing for sale.

Unbelievable breakthrough in recent research.

HOW? Four separate discoveries are combined in this new "cocktail" paradigm. Together they provide confirmed sweeping magic-bullet "cures" clinically tested and demonstrated to actually eliminate most "incurable" afflictions. _If you do it yourself you have nothing to buy except parts and batteries. Most have unconscious death-wishes manifested as disbelief, aversion, resistance and "defeat the unorthodox healer". But you must take back your own power and be willing to let go of your crutches._

What are the four easy protocols?

1. **_Blood Electrification:_** Microcurrents are known to eliminate all viruses, parasites, fungi, bacteria and pathogens in blood. Disclosed by many revolutionary patents and research over past years, these breakthroughs were lost or suppressed. The method was rediscovered by Einstein College of Medicine as an AIDS cure in 1990, then silenced.

2. **_Pulsed Kilogauss Magnetic Fields:_** Externally applied magnetic resonance of lymph, spleen, kidney & liver helps neutralize germinating, latent alien invaders and blocks re-infection. This quickens disease elimination, restores the immune system and supports detoxification. Permanent magnets, no matter how strong, will not nor can not scavenge pathogens with back-emf currents. You _must_ have a sharp time-varying, not DC, magnetic impulse.

3. **_Silver Colloids:_** Pennies-per-gallon self-made perfected colloids greatly assist in eliminating all known pathogens and guard against opportunistic infections. This "second immune system" is synergistic with steps 1, 2, and 4.

4. **_Drinking Ozonized Water:_** Rapid, safe, totally natural cell oxygenation without free radical damage. Universal detoxification by oxidation of wastes, dead and neutralized pathogens, (all anaerobic) reducing all to $H_2O + CO_2$ _without_ colonics, heat, liver and kidney flushing, herbs or other modalities. A low-cost, O_3 generator is fully described.

These four do-it-yourself tools are fully disclosed with detailed illustrated instructions for use. Utilized together and for two hours a day for about three weeks, they eliminate diseases. There is nothing to buy. No outside intervention, pharmaceuticals, herbs, enzymes or other treatments appear necessary. Some persons may need extra rest, liquids, trace minerals plus vitamins B and C during recovery. Malingerers justify avoidance by repeatedly demanding more "proof". If you show 100 cures, they'll insist on 1000, being more comfortable with peer approval than anything new.

Have these flour Proven cures been known previously? Apparently, but not in combination. Related discoveries have been reported in medical journals and patents over many years. Most were lost, ignored, disbelieved or suppressed by doctors and pharmaceutical cartels because this knowledge thwarts profiteering from people's suffering. US patents on related inventions establish public domain by prior state-of-the-art (many are pre-1982). Such miracle "cures" have been independently rediscovered and proven effective many times. Lately all four combined therapies were tested. This proved to be a synergistic breakthrough -the _magic-bullet_ solution to most diseases was found and confirmed by clinical studies including numerous PCR tests plus disappearance of all symptoms.

Why haven't doctors revealed this before now? _A patient cured is a medical customer lost!_ When actualized, these data could interrupt HMO profits; disrupt medical-pharmaceutical cartels; abort all biological warfare schemes; eliminate most drugs, medicines, debility, and early deaths; wipe out hospital and health care capital investments; minimize insurance machinations; dramatically abate sickness and suffering; plus imperil social security futures with bankruptcy; wreck sales of supplements, herbs, homeopathic and other health "remedies", machines, and practitioner's incomes. These are not politically correct.

It might permit a few _ethical_ practitioners to keep their Hippocratic oaths by giving back the patient's sovereignty instead of serving the AMA, FDA, and drug cartels. But this would decimate their incomes.

Bob Beck

Blood Electrification – The easy in-Vivo way

Revision May 16, 1997. Informational use only. Not intended as medical advice. Copyright © 1997 Robert C. Beck

Several years of experimentation and thousands of successes have resulted in simple, fast, proven ways to implement this most important step in self-healing.

1. Build your own or purchase a ready-to-use device, or put finishing touches on a nearly-completed kit available for $89 from Action Electronics, 1300 E. Edinger, Santa Ana, CA 92705. (714)-547-5169. With adequate detoxification, some use two or more blood electrifiers simultaneously to speed the recovery process, however one instrument works superbly.

2 Prepare and label a sea-salt-in-water solution for electrode wetting. Use ½ teaspoon of sea salt in a 2 ounce dropper bottle. Greater salt concentration can cause osmotic skin burns, irritation and rash. Add water and 4 drops of Pyrex or Clorox, Let salt dissolve. Filter through paper towel to clarify this storable conductive interface between cotton covered electrodes and skin. NEVER let bare metal electrode or any small area of metal touch skin directly, or it will burn. Use natural salt only, not table salt containing iodine for goiter end aluminum end silicates to insure easy pouring.

3. For best electrical conductance scrub skin at electrode locations with an alcohol swab or soap and water to eliminate oils, grime, dead cells, etc., rinse and dry. With fingertip rub a drop of salt water into pores along each electrode site.

4. Referring to illustrations, carefully feel for pulses and trace a line about 1 inch along at each wrist site precisely on top and inline (parallel) with located blood paths. Pulses are harder to feel on side opposite thumb. Never place electrodes over new lesions, cuts, abrasions, or sunburn. Muscle twitching in palm and fingers is normal and experienced occasionally.

5. Dip electrode covers into bottle to saturate initially. Position wet electrodes not over ~3/32 wide and 1-¼" long to wrist precisely over traced pulse paths. Slide from forearm side underneath a snug 1" wide stretch elastic band with Velcro holding overlapped ends. One electrode positions on radial (thumb) side, the second on opposite (ulnar) side of same hand. Current is confined to blood in lower forearm. Very little electrification is detectable elsewhere thus making safer for heart pacer users.

6. Put larger models in pocket and run electrode cord down sleeve or strap the smaller electrifier (single battery Sota instrument) with stretch-band to forearm. Plug in electrodes, turn on and advance slowly to comfortable level. The Sota is small, convenient, unobtrusive, uses one instead of three 9V batteries. Neither interferes with normal activities. (Sofa Instruments, PO Box 26161, Central Postal Station, Richmond, BC, Canada V6Y 3V3 1-(800)-224-0242).

7. Re-adjust power occasionally to maximum comfortable level. You can even sleep with it on without fear. When the treatment (about two hours per session daily for a month but only after detoxifying) is finished, turn it off and put it aside until tomorrow. Blood cleansing can be speeded with heat; example: wrapping forearm and hand with attached electrodes in heating pad set to high. When red and green LED's flash alternately with electrodes unplugged you know it's working properly.

8. Keep electrodes wet by re-moistening occasionally with drops of salt water using eye dropper in bottle cap. When finished rinse wrists. Wash electrodes periodically with soap, water and soft toothbrush to eliminate skin oils and soils. Soaking overnight will dissolve caked salt. Discoloration at ends is normal. When frayed or worn, discard old covers and rewrap stainless rods with 3 turns of 100% cotton flannel. Secure tightly with a few turns of thread wrapped to end, spiral back to beginning and tie. Electrodes should last for months, but wire leads break and must be replaced eventually.

What's inside the instruments? Preferred electrifiers must generate a 3.9 Hz (not critical) biphasic, 50% duty cycle sharp-rinse-time square wave, ± 27v peak adjustable output, capable of delivering several milliamperes into a low resistance load at skin surface (± 2000 Ω impedance) which after losses through tissue resistances delivers the necessary 50 to 100 microamperos through flowing blood. This suppressed medical discovery is proving to neutralize or eliminate all parasites and their mycotoxins, fungi, viruses, microbes, germs, pathogens, bacteria, or any other foreign invaders in blood without drugs. There are no known side effects to healthy cells, tissue, or fluids. Elimination can be verified by dark field / phase contrast microscopy.

Precautions: Badly debilitated patients such as full blown AIDS victims should begin electrification at less than 20 minutes every second day and flush by drinking lots of pure immediately-ozonized water because their systems will go into rapid detoxification causing physical symptoms called Herxheimer's syndrome. Users taking ANY medications, herbs, toxic vitamins or even *traces* of garlic in food should minimize these substances in blood for at least two days before starting and avoid other agents including coffee, tea, alcohol, tobacco, medications, recreational drugs, etc., during the several weeks of recovery. "Electroporation" is shown to increase dosage effects by levels up to 20 times normal of anything drunk, shot, or ingested thus causing problems. This is documented by J.C. Weaver, Harvard-MIT, *Journal of Cellular Biochemistry*, 51: 426-435;1993. Patients needing essential medications should take them immediately after turning off electrification and wait 24 hours before next blood cleansing. This lets drug residues decay to minimum levels in plasma before re-electrifying. If detoxing becomes disturbing, proceed even more slowly. Symptoms may include fever, giddiness, dizziness, headaches, light-headed vagueness, nausea, skin rashes, eruptions, itching, boils; coughing, kidney and liver discomfort, aches, general malaise, inflammations, frequent urination, and sluggishness. Use caution when detoxing patents with impaired liver or kidney function. But remember it's far better to force wastes out of your system than leaving stored where they may have been hiding for years.

Treat even more slowly if initial discomfort occurs. Electrification will profoundly improve your health and sometimes provoke your deepest unconscious mind-sets such as everyone's conflicting guilt and death wishes. This generally causes noticeable anxiety and depression which may accompany recoveries.

Bob Beck

OZONE REVISITED

Offered for Educational and Informational Purposes Only; not Intended as Medical Advice

Preliminary data May 13, 1997 Copyright © 1997 Robert C. Beck

Recent re-evaluation of ozone suggests that while it is controversial as a stand-alone therapy, O^3 when directly ingested in water simultaneously with electroporation (biphasic microcurrents in arteries) provides a truly remarkable boost to total system oxygenation, *plus natural and rapid detoxification*. Measurements show dramatic increases in blood oxygen within minutes using meters like the Nellcor® NPB-40 "Percent Oxygen Saturation Meter" [Nellcor Puritan Bennett, Inc., Pleasanton, CA 94599, 1-800-NELLCOR]. Many different "Ozonizers sold at health expos for *prices up to $4700* are large heavy suitcases, must plug into AC, and almost universally use vastly inferior *Ultra-Violet* systems and bottled oxygen instead of the preferred high-voltage cold-corona utilizing *air* for ozone production. Described here is a superior design producing faster, more concentrated O^3 than other available home units. It is a very portable three-way, stand-alone system. You can choose to utilize either internal battery power, or AC plug-in, or car lighter powered input. It can be put together by anyone for a fraction of the cost of top-of-the-line ozonizers. A second cheaper but slower do-it-yourself design using AC power only is also shown here. It uses inexpensive parts for the budget-minded but still works superbly. O^3 unlike other forms of oxygen carries *negative* electrical charges that specifically counteract free radical damages, scavenge crosslinking and re-charge depleted cells. Ionic silver colloids also greatly assist this "rejuvenation" process by restoring free electrons.

O^3 rapidly converts (oxidizes) all known toxins and wasts long present in your body cells to H_2O and CO_2 which flush out easily and rapidly without utilizing colonics, lymph, spleen, liver, or kidney detoxing or any other treatments.

BUILDING A COMPACT, LINE-DEPENDENT AC/DC LOW COST POWERFUL OZONE GENERATOR USING AIR AND NOT REQUIRING EXPENSIVE BOTTLED OXYGEN

Connect together in this order

1- 12.6 V-1.2 Ampere-hour rechargeable lead-acid gel-cell battery (~1-½ hr./charge)	$ 16.50
1- In-line fuse holder (EM brand GMA 18 Ga.)	2.49
1- 5- 8 Amp short fuses; Female spade .187, 18-22 GA battery connectors	3.15
Action Electronics, 1300 E. Edinger Ave., Santa Ana, CA 92705 (714) 547-5169	
1- Connector set, cigarette lighter male plug and female jack.	2.50
1- 12V dc to 110V ac inverter (*NOTEpower* brand, model #PW-50)	71.95
Mar Vac Electronics, 2001 Harbor, Costa Mesa, CA 92627 (714) 645-6448	
1- AC adapter to triple outlet (Drugstore)	~2.00
1- Aquarium aerification pump (Schego Optimal 5 W 250 liter/hour membrane)	35.00
Strictly Fish, 12227 Harbor Blvd., Garden Grove, CA (714) 750-7151	
1- German Sander brand model 200 fish tank ozonizer, adjustable 0-200 mg O^3	389.00
TIS Tropical Fish, 16175 Brookhurst, Fountain Valley, CA (714) 839-1740	
1- 25ft. flexible plastic airline tubing ¼" OD cat. #14507	3.89
1- Check Valve (prevents water from back-siphoning into ozonizer)	2.19
1- Airstone (glass bead or ceramic - not plastic) Fine bubbles, Kordon #62503	2.49
1- (Optional) Spring-wound timer, 0-60 min. or SPST. switch (*Fry's Electronics*)	12.00
Switch cuts off system at selected time. Wire between battery and inverter	
You may need a plastic, leather, or canvas bag or other small carrying case.	
Total: Retail price for currently preferred system: (Only $324.00 wholesale.)	**$ 540.50**

A less expensive but excellent system is described next. It plugs into 115V AC, uses less powerful and fewer parts, is somewhat slower, but produces the highest quality ozone from ambient air or bottled oxygen.

1- Sander model 25 hi-voltage cold-corona aquarium ozonizer.	$ 169.99
1- Whisper #500 aquarium air pump; Silaflex II (not rubber) diphragm & valves.	26.99
Fishland, 13079 Harbor Blvd., Garden Grove, CA 92643	
Misc., plastic tubing, check valve, fine bubble stone, extension cord, etc.	8.60
Total: *Retail cost for complete system. (Only $123.35 Wholesale)*	**$ 205.58**

List prices: Sander Ozonizers 25 mg-$169.99; 50 mg-$189.99; 100 mg-$244.99; and 200 mg (most powerful "portable") for $389.00 Purchase the strongest corona unit you can afford. Avoid cheaper, weaker Ultra-Violet types.

Note: Nitrogen by-products, oxides and acids produced with *air* and *cold corona* discharge have been tested and found negligible and harmless in ozonized drinking water. But *hot arcing* produces unwanted byproducts using air; pure oxygen does not. So to be safe start with *bottled* oxygen and pure water only if making O³ intended for inter-muscular injection, insufflation, direct blood infusions, or with heparin for auto-dialysis (bubbling blood in a vessel for re-injection or "autohemotherapy"). "Medical" & "Industrial" (welding) oxygen are *identical* and come from the same tanks at suppliers who charge more by pretending that "medical-grade" oxygen is somehow "different". Ambient air works well for drinkable O³. The colder and purer your water and the deeper the container for greater pressure plus the smaller the volume of H³O being bubbled, the most ozone dissolves faster and the longer it lasts. Ideal bubblers are ~3" dia. X 2-½ ft. high Teflon or Polypropylene tubes with airstone at very bottom. Tall, thin plastic bottles work almost as well but their greater content takes a little longer for saturation. Non-reactive Pyrex containers are better.

To use: submerge airstone to *bottom* and "bubble" ~10 OZ containers of ½ ice + ½ cold tap water for ~5 minutes with the inexpensive design or ~2 min. with the more powerful 200 mg ozonizer. Charge *cold* water in a large bottle for ~25 min. Drink immediately since O⁹ without stabilizers even in ice water has a half-life of about 20 minutes so retains full potency for only a short time. Benefits start in minutes and are far superior to many other expensive products claimed to provide "bound" oxygen (chlorites; ClO²) or proprietary "Vitamin O" stabilized oxygen boosters. Ozone cannot be stored which is why everyone needs his own generator to make O⁹ immediately before using for the best possible results.

Never breathe ozone or ozonized air as it damages (oxidizes) lung tissue even in small quantities.

Bob Beck

Ozone Revisited

— process flow diagram for making your own ozonated water

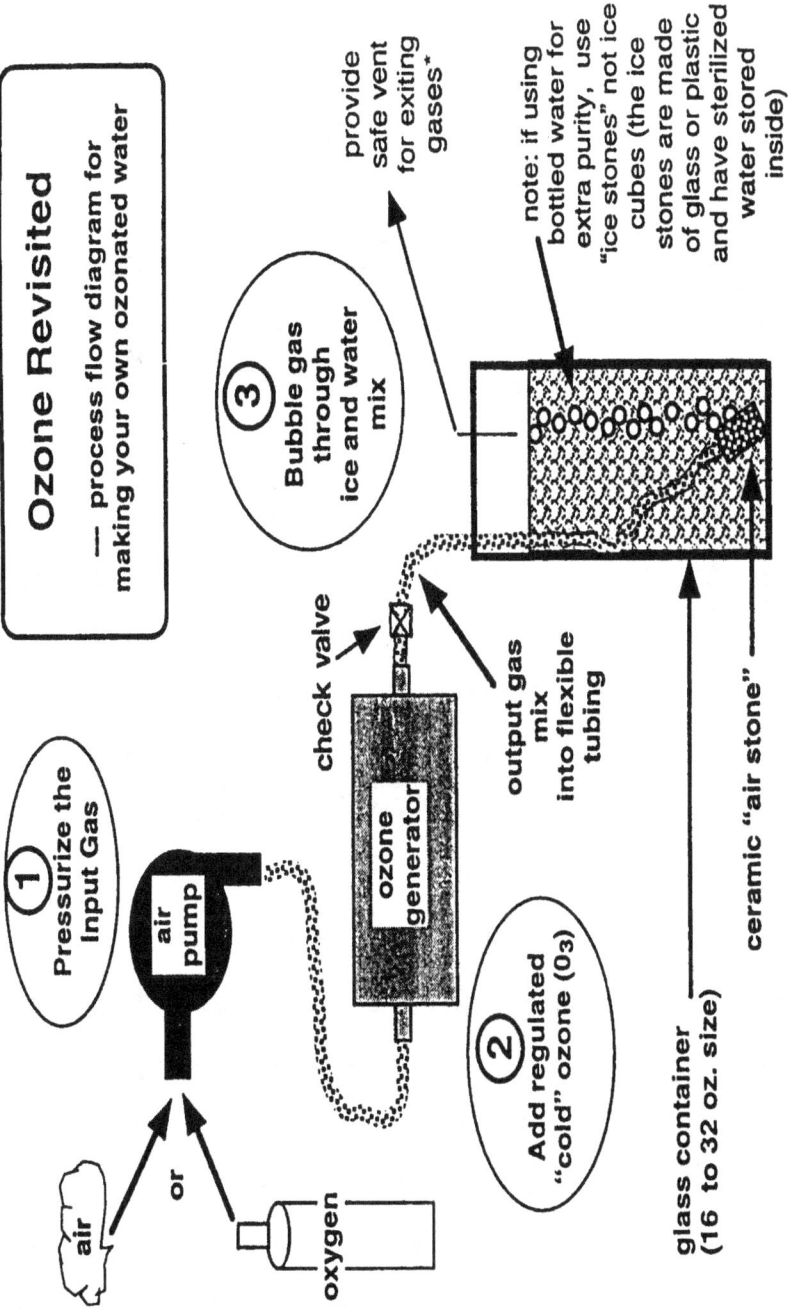

① Pressurize the Input Gas

air

or

oxygen

air pump

② Add regulated "cold" ozone (O3)

ozone generator

check valve

output gas mix into flexible tubing

③ Bubble gas through ice and water mix

provide safe vent for exiting gases*

note: if using bottled water for extra purity, use "ice stones" not ice cubes (the ice stones are made of glass or plastic and have sterilized water stored inside)

glass container (16 to 32 oz. size)

ceramic "air stone"

④ **Finally, set process timer**

(controls O_3 bubbling time, as from
2 to 5 minutes. see text for details)

→ Note: always drink or use ozonated water
within 20 minutes after making.

*Caution: do _not_ breath in ozonated gas... (the
chemical activation that gives it power to cleanse is too
strong for lung tissue and can easily cause damage)

NEW PERIODIC TABLE
Revised 1995

1 H 1.00797	2 He 4.0026	3 Li 6.939	4 Be 9.0122	5 B 10.811	6 C 12.01115	7 N 14.0067	8 O 15.9994	9 F 18.9984	10 Ne 20.183	11 Na 22.98977	12 Mg 24.312
13 Al 26.98154	14 Si 28.0855	15 P 30.97376	16 S 32.064	17 Cl 35.453	18 Ar 39.948	19 K 39.0983	20 Ca 40.08	21 Sc 44.9559	22 Ti 47.90	23 V 50.9414	24 Cr 51.996
25 Mn 54.9380	26 Fe 55.847	27 Co 58.9332	28 Ni 58.71	29 Cu 63.546	30 Zn 65.37	31 Ga 69.72	32 Ge 72.59	33 As 74.9216	34 Se 78.96	35 Br 79.904	36 Kr 83.80
37 Rb 85.4678	38 Sr 87.62	39 Y 88.9059	40 Zr 91.22	41 Nb 92.9054	42 Mo 95.94	43 Tc (97)	44 Ru 101.07	45 Rh 102.9055	46 Pd 106.4	47 Ag 107.868	48 Cd 112.40
49 In 114.82	50 Sn 118.69	51 Sb 121.75	52 Te 127.60	53 I 126.9044	54 Xe 131.30	55 Cs 132.9054	56 Ba 137.33	57 La 138.9055	58 Ce 140.12	59 Pr 140.9077	60 Nd 144.24

61 **Pm** (145)	62 **Sm** 150.35	63 **Eu** 151.96	64 **Gd** 157.25	65 **Tb** 158.9254	66 **Dy** 162.50	67 **Ho** 164.9304	68 **Er** 167.26	69 **Tm** 168.9342	70 **Yb** 173.04	71 **Lu** 174.97	72 **Hf** 178.49
73 **Ta** 180.9479	74 **W** 183.85	75 **Re** 186.207	76 **Os** 190.2	77 **Ir** 192.22	78 **Pt** 195.09	79 **Au** 196.9665	80 **Hg** 200.59	81 **Tl** 204.37	82 **Pb** 207.19	83 **Bi** 208.9804	84 **Po** (209)
85 **At** (210)	86 **Rn** (222)	87 **Fr** (223)	88 **Ra** 226.0254	89 **Ac** (227)	90 **Th** 232.0381	91 **Pa** 231.0359	92 **U** 238.029	93 **Np** 237.0482	94 **Pu** (244)	95 **Am** (243)	96 **Cm** (247)
97 **Bk** (247)	98 **Cf** (251)	99 **Es** (254)	100 **Fm** (257)	101 **Md** (258)	102 **No** (259)	103 **Lr** (260)	104 **Ku** (260)	105 **Ha** (260)	106 — (263)	107 — (280)	108 — (288)
109 — (296)	110 — (296)	111 **Pe** (292)	112 **Dk** (300)	113 **Cb** (299)	114 **Ci** (302)	115 **Ab** (305)	116 **Im** (305)	117 **To** (306)	118 **Zi** (318)	119 **Dd** (315)	120 **Rd** (314)
121 **Bo** (317)	122 **Db** (319)	123 **Mu** (320)	124 **It** 3.22	125 **Ro** (333)	126 **Tn** (323)	127 **Tv** (328)	128 **Tt** (328)	129 **Tr** (332)	139 **Ki** (348)	140 **Ct** (361)	

Note: Numbers in parentheses indicate the mass number with the most stable isotope, (good enough for our civilization at the moment). Shading indicates elements of Alien origin.

Blood Electrification - Reprint of Patent # 5,188,738

United States Patent 5,188,738 Kaali, et. al. * Feb. 23, 1993

Alternating current supplied electrically conductive method and system for treatment of blood and/or other body fluids and/or synthetic fluids with electric forces.

Inventors: Kaali; Steven (88 Ashford Ave., Dobbs Ferry, NY 10522); Schwolsky; Peter M. (4101 Cathedral Ave., NW., Washington, DC 20016). [*] Notice: The portion of the term of this patent subsequent to Aug. 18, 2009 has been disclaimed. Appl. No.: 615,437 Filed: Nov. 16, 1990

Related U.S. Application Data

Continuation-in-part of Ser No. 562,721, Aug. 6, 1990, abandoned.Intl. Cl.: B01D 35//06 A61K 41/00 U.S. Cl.: 210/748; 128/419.R: 128/421; 128/783; 128/784; 204/131; 204/164; 204/186; 204/302; 210/243; 422/ 22; 422/ 44; 604/ 4 Field of Search: 210/243, 748, 764; 128/419 R, 421, 783, 784; 604/4: 422/22, 44; 204/131,164, 186, 242, 275, 302, 305

References Cited

U.S. Patent Documents

592,735	Oct., 1897	Jones	204/242
672,231	Apr., 1901	Lacomme	204/275
2,490,730	Dec., 1949	Dubilier	204/305
3,692,648	Sept., 1972	Matloff et al.	204/129
3,753,886	Aug., 1973	Myers	204/186
3,878,564	Apr., 1975	Yao et al.	210/648
3,965,008	Jun., 1976	Dawson	422/ 22
3,994,799	Nov., 1976	Yao et al.	210/321.64
4,473,449	Sept., 1984	Michaels et al.	204/101
4,616,640	Oct., 1986	Kaali et al.	128/130
4,770,167	Sept., 1988	Kaali et al.	128/788
4,932,421	Jun., 1990	Kaali et al.	128/831
5,049,252	Sept., 1991	Murrell	210/243
5,058,065	Oct., 1991	Slovak	128/783
5,133,932	Jul., 1992	Gunn et al.	210/748

Foreign Patent Documents

995848   Jul., 1983   SU   210/243

Other References

Proceedings of the Society for Experimental Biology & Medicine, vol.1, (1979), pp. 204-209, "Inactivation of Herpes Simples Virus with Methylene Blue, Light and Electricity"—Mitchell R. Swartz et al.

Journal of the Clinical Investigation published by the American Society for Clinical Investigations, Inc., vol. 65, Feb. 1980, pp. 432-438--"Mechanisms of Photodynamic Inactivation of Herpes Simplex Viruses"—Lowell E. Schnipper et al.

Journal of Clinical Microbiology, vol. 17, No. 2, Feb. 1983, pp. 374-376, "Photodynamic Inactivation of Pseudorabier Virus with Methylene Blue Dye, Light and Electricity"—Janine A. Badyisk et al.

Primary Examiner: Dawson; Robert A.
Assistant Examiner: Kim; Sun Uk Attorney, Agent or Firm: Charles W. Helzer

Abstract

A new alternating current process and system for treatment of blood and/or other body fluids and/or synthetic fluids from a donor to a recipient or storage receptacle or in a recycling system using novel electrically conductive treatment vessels for treating blood and/or other body fluids and/or synthetic fluids with electric field forces of appropriate electric field strength to provide electric current flow through the blood or other body fluids at a magnitude that is biologically compatible but is sufficient to render the bacteria, virus, parasites and/or fungus ineffective to infect or affect normally healthy cells while maintaining the biological usefulness of the blood or other fluids. For this purpose low voltage alternating current electric potentials are applied to the treatment vessel which are of the order of from about 0.2 to 12 volts and produce current flow densities in the blood or other fluids of from one microampere per square millimeter of electrode area exposed to the fluid being treated t about two milliamperes per square millimeter.

31 Claims, 26 Drawing Figures

This invention relates to novel electrically conductive methods and systems employing electrically conductive vessels provided with electrically conductive surfaces for use in subjecting blood and/or other body fluids and/or synthetic fluids such as tissue culture medium to direct treatment by alternating current electric forces.

BACKGROUND PROBLEM

It is now well known in the medical profession and the general public that blood collected in a blood bank from a large number of donors may be contaminated by contaminants such as bacteria, virus, parasites and/or fungus obtained from even a single donor. While screening of donors has done much to alleviate this problem, the screening of donors can and does miss occasional donors whose blood is unfit for use. When this occurs and the unfit blood is mixed with otherwise usable blood, the entire batch must be discarded for transfusion purposes. Because of this problem, the present invention has been devised to attenuate any bacteria, virus (including the AIDS HIV virus) parasites and/or fungus contained in blood contributed by a donor to the point that any such contaminant is rendered ineffective for infecting a normally healthy human cell, but does not make the blood biologically unfit for use in humans. Similar problems exist with respect to treatment of other body fluids, such as amniotic fluids. The treatent method and system is also applicable to mammals other than humans.

In addition to the above, there is a need for methods and systems for the treatment of blood and/or other body fluids both in in-situ processing wherein the treated blood and/or other body fluids are withdrawn from the body, treated and then returned to the body in a closed loop, recirculating treatment process that is located near but outside the patient's body, or the treatment can be effected through implanted treatment system components.

In co-pending United States application serial No. 07/615,800 entitled "Electrically Conductive Methods and Systems for Treatment of Blood and Other Body Fluids with Electric Forces"-Steven Kaali and Peter M. Schwolsky, inventors, filed concurrently and co-pending with this application, a similar treatment method and system employing direct current excitation potentials is described and claimed. The disclosure of co-pending application Ser. No. 07/615,800 hereby is incorporated into this application in its entirety.

SUMMARY OF INVENTION

The present invention provides new electrically conductive methods and systems using alternating electric current excitation potentials for treating blood and/or other body fluids, such as amniotic fluids, and/or synthetic fluids such as tissue culture medium from a donor to a transfusion recipient or to a storage receptacle, or for recirculating a single donor's or patient's blood or other body fluids. The treatment can be accomplished in a treatment system external of the body or by implant devices for purging contaminants using a novel electrically conductive vessel for direct electric treatment of blood or other body fluids, such as amniotic fluids, with alternating current electric field forces of appropriate electric field strength to attenuate such contaminants to the extent that bacteria, virus, fungus, and/or parasites contained in the blood or other body fluids are rendered ineffective to infect and/or affect normally healthy human cells. The treatment, however, does not render the blood or other body fluids biologically unfit for use in humans or other mammals after the treatment. The new methods and systems according to the invention achieve these ends without requiring time consuming and expensive processing procedures and equipment in addition to those normally required in the handling of blood or other body fluids or synthetic fluids. The invention can be used to achieve the electric field force treatment during the normally occurring transfer processing from a donor to a recipient or to a collection receptacle, or recirculation of a single donor's or patient's blood or other body fluids, such as amniotic fluids.

What Does Beck's Work Mean-Theoretically?

Beck's work establishes **Energetics** as an incredible shift in the 21st century health paradigm![1] Not only that, he has publicized that fact that in 1993, the United States Patent Office certified that the medical device, patent number 5188738, *"will attenuate [breakdown] any bacteria or virus (including AIDS/HIV), parasites and all fungi contained in the blood, rendering them ineffective from infecting a normally healthy human cell."* Hence, <u>**we must conclude that the United States government, and many in the medical community, have known of an inexpensive and effective method for arresting HIV since the 1990s.**</u>[2]

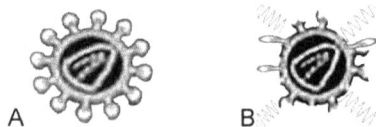

Image A represents a healthy virus. Image B represents the same virus after blood electrification.

---

[1] The transformation from impersonal industrial control to safer personal control over one's own health! (See page 190)
[2] Global Sciences Congress: <u>THE BOB BECK INTERVIEW</u>
The fact that Beck was <u>**NO MOUSE CHASING CHEESE**</u> has benefited mankind inestimably!!!

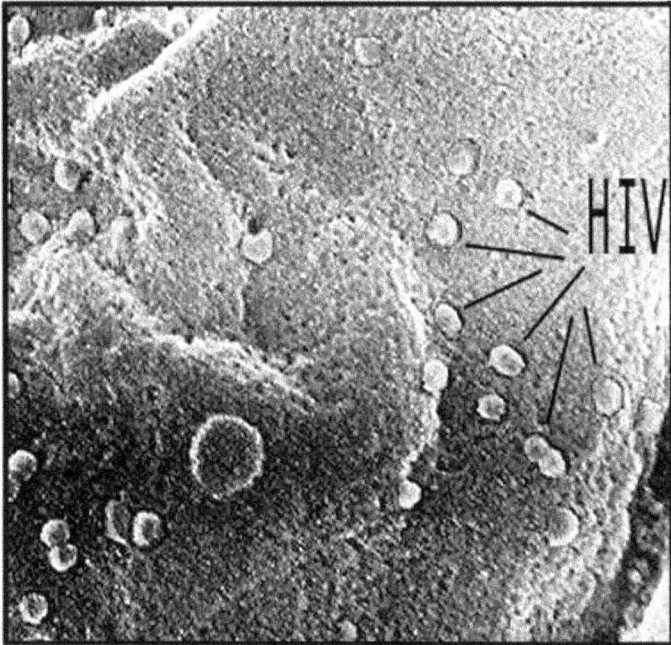

HIV is the virus that causes AIDS. Millions die from AIDS each year. Energy therapy has been proven to arrest this virus with no harmful side-effects!

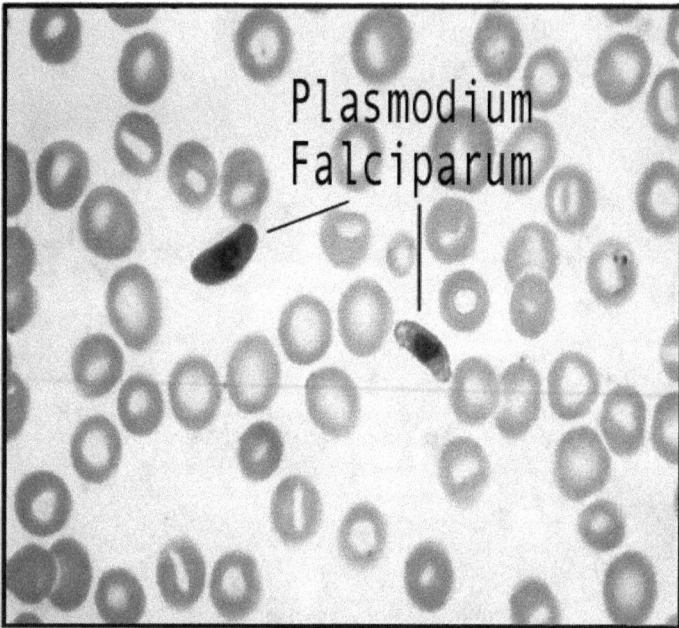

This is the Malaria parasite. Millions die from Malaria each year. Energy therapy has been proven to arrest this parasite with no harmful side-effects!

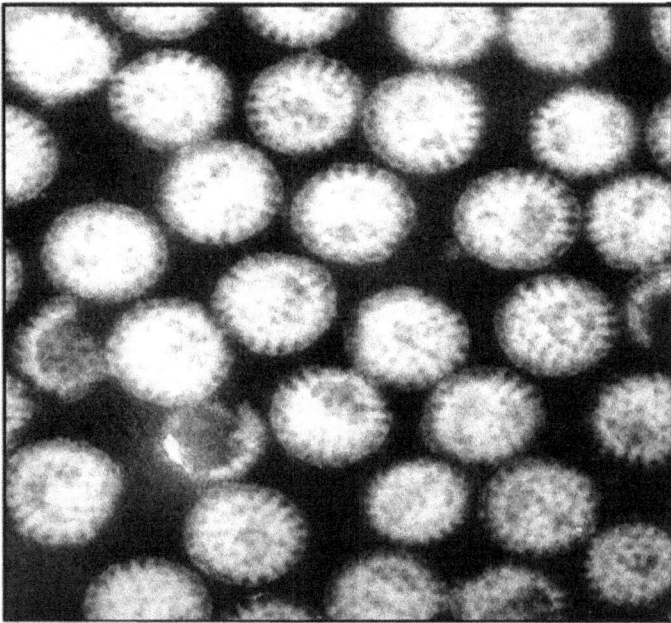

*These are Rotavirus particles.
Millions die from Diarrhea
each year. Energy therapy
has been proven to arrest this
virus with no harmful side-effects!*

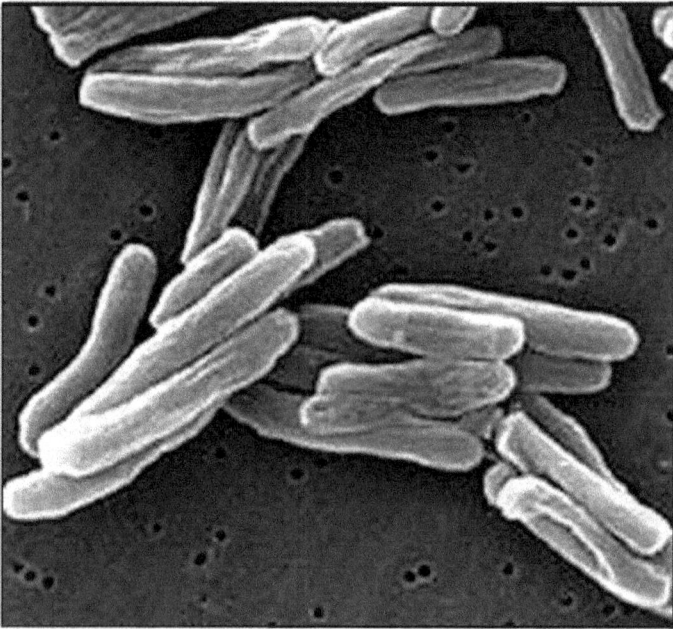

This is Mycobacterium. Millions die from Tuberculosis each year. Energy therapy has been been proven to arrest this bacteria with no harmful side-effects!

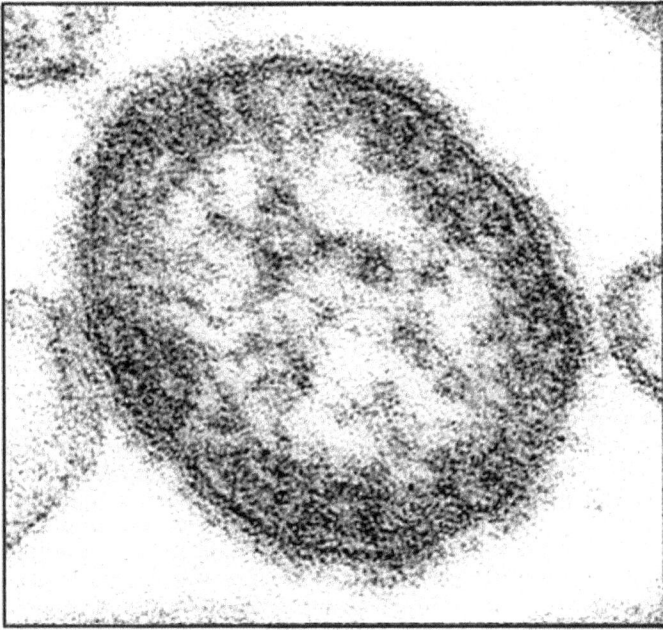

Paramyxoviruses cause Measles. A half-million die from this illness each year. Energy therapy has been proven to arrest this virus with no harmful side-effects!

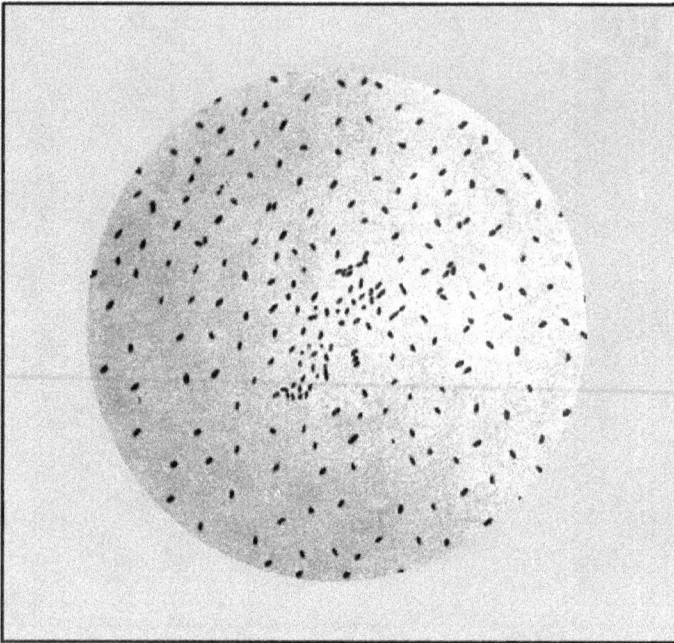

This is Bordetella pertussis. It is the bacteria which causes Whopping Cough. Hundreds of thousands die from this illness each year. Energy therapy has been proven to arrest this organism with no harmful side-effects!

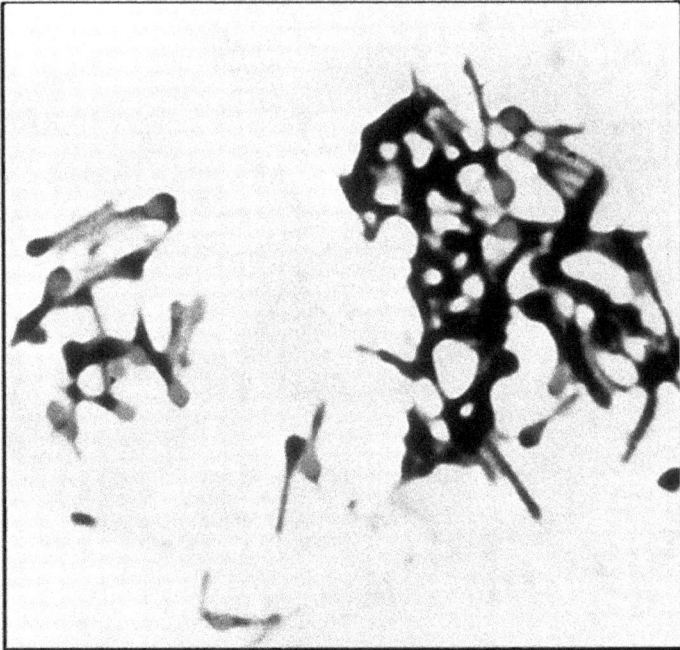

This is Clostridium tetani. It is the bacteria which causes Tetanus. Hundreds of thousands die from this illness each year. Energy therapy has been proven to arrest this organism with no harmful side-effects!

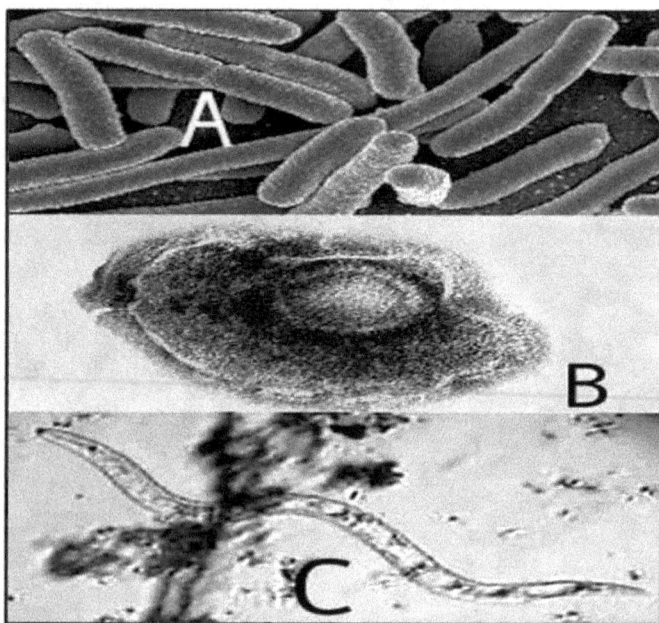

Meningitis can be caused by bacteria, viruses and/or parasites. For example: A – E. coli bacteria; B – Varicella virus; C – Roundworm parasite. Tens of thousands die from this illness each year. Energy therapy has been proven to arrest such microorganisms with no harmful side-effects!

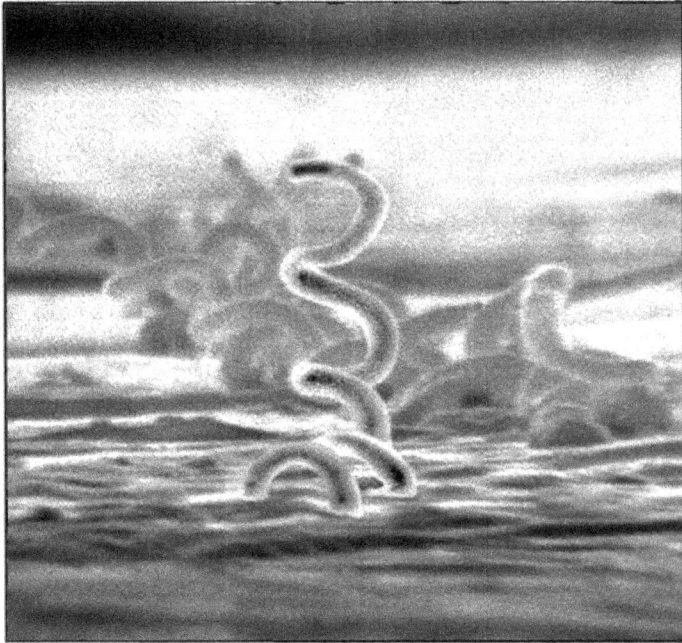

This is Treponema pallidum. It is the cause of syphilis. Tens of thousands die from this illness each year. Energy therapy has been proven to arrest this bacteria with no harmful side-effects!

These are some of the deadliest killers on the planet; and in truth, we could go on and on like this. <u>The reason is because microcurrents are devastating to **All** microorganisms—and blood electrification is the application of such</u>![3] We are all greatly indebted to the physicist from California, who came to use his expertise in low-level electromagnetic energy to heal for free, as opposed to mischief for a price.

Before closing, there is one more area that I would like to touch upon—**<u>Vaccination</u>**. Each year, legal FDA approved vaccines harm a large number of people.[4] While the causes for harm are no doubt varied, if pathogenic microorganisms injected into my body were a concern of mine—*I would investigate Energetics and the Beck Protocol stat.* Furthermore, in theory, this could be doubly important in the case of children because of their tremendous recuperative abilities.

---

[3] **<u>All means natural and manmade microorganisms</u>**.
[4] Horowitz, L., <u>Emerging Viruses and Vaccinations</u> & (See page 188)

What Does This Mean— Theoretically?

In Becker and Seldon's <u>The Body Electric</u>, we find the following:

> *"The amputation of a fingertip—by a car-door, lawnmower, electric fan, or whatever—is one of the most common childhood injuries. The standard treatment is to smooth the exposed bone and stitch the skin closed, or, if the digit has been retrieved and was cleanly cut, to try to reattach it by microsurgery. The sad fact is that even the most painstaking surgery gives less than optimal results . . . In the early 70s at the emergency room of Sheffield Children's Hospital in England, one youngster with such an injury benefited from a clerical mixup . . . the customary referral to a surgeon was never made. When the error was caught a few days later, surgeon Cynthia Illingworth noticed that the fingertip was regenerating! She merely watched nature take its course . . . by 1974 she'd documented several hundred*

re-grown fingertips, all in children 11 years old or younger."[5]

Insomuch as young children are *teeming* with life, there may be no limit (*in the case of injury due to microbial infection*) to the body's regenerative capabilities, once the offending organisms have been attenuated or removed—THEORETICALLY . . .

O' yeah, before I forget—if you're waiting for CNN, Fox or the AMA to sanction Energetics for the herd—don't hold your breath. America's Medical Industrial Complex charges hundreds of thousands of dollars for every cancer patient; and tens of thousands for other illnesses like AIDS. Conversely, the hypothetical cost of using Energetics to treat such patients would probably be well under a thousand dollars.[6]

---

[5] Becker, R., & Seldon, G., The Body Electric pp. 155 - 156
[6] The Granada Forum: Suppressed Medical Discovery DVD
Beck was fond of saying—*Disease-causing microbes could be eliminated from the blood for the price of a pack of gum!*

What Does This Mean— Theoretically?

United States Patent [19]

Kaali et al.

[11] Patent Number: 5,185,086

[45] Date of Patent: Feb. 9, 1993

US005185086A

[54] METHOD AND SYSTEM FOR TREATMENT
OF BLOOD AND/OR OTHER BODY FLUIDS
AND/OR SYNTHETIC FLUIDS USING
COMBINED FILTER ELEMENTS AND
ELECTRIC FIELD FORCES

[76] Inventors: **Steven Kaali**, 88 Ashford Ave.,
Dobbs Ferry, N.Y. 10522; **Peter M.
Schwolsky**, 20 Haslet Ave.,
Princeton, N.J. 08540

[21] Appl. No.: **730,690**

[22] Filed: **Jul. 16, 1991**

[51] Int. Cl.^{5} **B01D 35/06; B01D 37/00;
A61K 41/00**

[52] U.S. Cl. **210/748; 55/487;
128/419 R; 128/421; 128/783; 204/131;
204/164; 204/186; 204/302; 210/243; 210/251;
210/314; 210/335; 210/416.1; 210/472;
210/634; 422/22; 422/44; 422/101**

[58] Field of Search 210/748, 764, 767, 243,
210/500.1, 498, 251, 314, 335, 641, 645, 650,
651, 634, 472, 258, 416.1; 55/483, 488; 128/419
R, 421, 783, 784; 604/4; 422/22, 44, 101;
204/131, 186, 164, 242, 275, 302, 305, 264, 276,
235

[56]   **References Cited**

U.S. PATENT DOCUMENTS

2,428,328   9/1947   Ham et al. 204/186

3,398,082	8/1968	Lochmann et al.	204/302
3,753,886	8/1973	Myers	204/186
3,980,541	9/1976	Aine	204/302
4,303,530	12/1981	Shah et al.	210/489
4,473,449	9/1984	Michaels et al.	210/748
4,594,138	6/1986	Thompson	204/302
4,751,003	6/1988	Raehse et al.	210/641
4,800,011	1/1989	Abbott et al.	210/748
5,076,933	12/1991	Glenn et al.	210/335
5,085,773	2/1992	Danowski	210/243
5,133,352	7/1992	Lathrop et al.	128/419 R
5,139,684	8/1992	Kaali et al.	210/243

Primary Examiner—Robert A. Dawson
Assistant Examiner—Sun Uk Kim
Attorney, Agent, or Firm—Charles W. Helzer

[57]   **ABSTRACT**

A method and system for the treatment of blood and/or
other body fluids (such as amniotic fluids) as well as
synthetic fluids such as tissue culture medium whereby
a fluid to be treated is mechanically filtered for elimination of particles contained therein which exceed 0.2
microns in size (or some other minutely small size) and
in addition subjecting the fluid being treated to electric
field forces in the microwatt/milliwatt region induced
by relatively low voltage of a few volts and low current
density which does not exceed values which could
impair the biological usefulness and characteristics of
the blood or other fluid being treated.

19 Claims, 1 Drawing Sheet

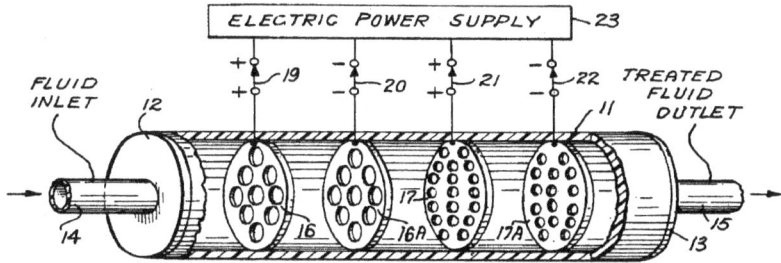

**Despite denials by academics, health professionals
and an assortment of other MIC lackeys—this
diagram is of the United States patent for 5,185,086.
Issued on February 9, 1993, this patent (*just one of
several*) completely validates the scientific principle
of microcurrents attenuating microorganisms! Bob
Beck would later improve on the execution of the
science with his in vivo (rather than in vitro) device
and procedures.[7]**

---

[7] Bob Beck Lecture: Take Back Your Power

Conversation
with an Energy
Practitioner

Conversation with an Energy Therapist

IN THE COURSE OF MY RESEARCH FOR THIS BOOK, I HAVE HAD A NUMBER OF CONVERSATIONS WITH PEOPLE WHO'VE UNDERGONE ALLOPATHIC TREATMENTS FOR A WIDE RANGE OF ILLNESSES. DURING THIS INVESTIGATION, BY SHEER HAPPEN-STANCE, I MET AN ELDERLY GENTLEMAN WHO HAD ACTUALLY BEEN AN ENERGY PRACTITIONER FOR SEVERAL YEARS. COMPLETELY AMAZED BY WHAT HE TOLD—I ASKED HIS PERMISSION TO SHARE SOME OF HIS STORY WITH YOU. I HAVE TAKEN THE LIBERTY OF CONDENSING OUR TALKS INTO ONE BRIEF DISCUSSION. I WANT TO SHARE IT BECAUSE ON SEVERAL OCCASIONS—OVER A PERIOD OF MONTHS—HIS STORY REMAINED CONSTANT, AND I HAVE COME ACROSS OTHER INDEPENDENT INFORMATION WHICH SUPPORTS HIS TESTIMONY! HIS NAME HAS BEEN CHANGED HERE TO PROTECT HIS PRIVACY. ONCE MORE, <u>THIS INFORMATION IS INTENDED FOR RESEARCH AND/OR THEORETICAL PURPOSES—AND NOT TO BE SEEN AS MEDICAL ADVICE</u> . . .

ENERGETICS

After hundreds of random encounters with people who have major health concerns—one rainy morning I met a gentleman (whom I shall call) Walter. Here is a portion of our conversation.

RL:
How long have you been living in Seattle?

Walter:
I just moved here. I use to live in _____. (*I am not going to reveal the state; suffice it to say its in the Western United States.*)

RL:
What were you doing there?

Walter:
I retired as a civil service employee a while back.

RL:
How do you like Seattle?

Walter:
I like the area I live in, but at my age, the weather really affects me.

RL:
Do you mean the cold and the rain?

Walter:
That's right. It is much hotter and dryer in ____, and I really miss my ionizer. I put it in storage when moved up here to be closer to my daughter.

RL:
I've never heard of an ionizer—what is that?

Walter:
It is a machine that ionizes parts of the body.

RL:
You said machine; do you mean a plugging it into a wall socket, and turning it on type of device?

Walter:
It is an electrical device; but you don't plug it into an AC wall outlet—it runs on a 6-volt DC battery.

Let me stop and say that this was the beginning of my curiosity about ionization. Whenever I saw Walter, we'd eventually get back to talking about his experiences ionizing. And in every case, he would satisfy me that he had a great deal of knowledge and experience in this field!

RL:
When did you first begin to ionize?

Walter:
Around 30-years ago.

RL:
So, how did you learn about it?

Walter:
A friend got me a job at a racetrack, and the horse trainers there were using ionizers on the injured horses. That's where I first learned about it.

RL:
I see.

Walter:
There was a powerful Arabian horse named ____ that was used in the film ____ (*a very popular big budget movie*). One day, he reared up and came down so hard that he fractured his shoulder horribly. It was so serious that he might have been put down—but we used the ionizer and the bones eventually regenerated enough to save the shoulder and allow him to have a normal life!

RL:
How long did the process take?

Walter:

It took quite a while, but he was an agreeable horse, so the shoulder eventually got better.

RL:
That's incredible. I have met a lot of sick and injured people but I've never heard of an ionizer before today. There is such a disconnect between what's possible and what's widely known.

Walter:
I'll say: we used it on hundreds of horses with fractures, strains and breaks. A hairline fracture would normally heal up after a couple of months—**with the ionizer we could accelerate that to about two-weeks**!

RL:
I wonder if it would work that way on humans?

Walter:
My daughter hurt her shoulder and she used the ionizer. Not only did it help her shoulder, but it also got rid of a cold she had.

RL:
That means it also fights microorganisms; did you use it for infections on the horses too?

Walter:

Yes—on many occasions, and with good results!

RL:
Remarkable.

Walter:
Have you heard of Secretariat?

RL:
Sure.

Walter:
Secretariat got infected with laminitis; ultimately he was put down. But in my opinion, ionizing would have stopped his infection.

RL:
Did you ever work on Secretariat?

Walter:
No. Secretariat was a horse out of the East.

RL:
Too bad his trainer didn't know about your work with ionizing.

Walter:
Every trainer has their own beliefs about the best way to take care of their horses.

RL:
Seems like everyone would have been happy to have you guys on call—as long as they could afford you.

Walter:
You'd be surprised. If you charge someone a lot for something, they want you more than if you are reasonable. And we didn't charge very much.

RL:
Unbelievable: What you just said is, *"If you're not a crook—I don't want to deal with you—even if you're helping me and giving me a good deal!"*

Walter:
Yep.

RL:
Were the people at your track the only people you know who used ionizers on their horses?

Walter:
No. But everyone didn't get the same results because every horse is different. Our results were good because we were adept at it!

RL:
What do you mean when you say every horse is different?

Walter:
The ionizer produces a sensation; *some horses will get frightened and bolt.*

RL:
I see. I wonder why ionizing isn't used in hospitals?

Walter:
Some probably do, but under different terminology. I think that the machine I used in the 80s was bought from the company that made it by a team of doctors.

RL:
You'd think they'd be using it in a lot of areas by now . . .

While Walt went on for hours discussing training prizewinning horses and his life in the Western U.S., I will stop here.

Dear researchers you are free to embrace, or reject, this information. I must say that in all of the time I spent with Walt, I never had occasion to think that he was doing anything other than relating the truth about his experiences. Let me close with some periphery evidence that lends credence to his story.

Walter gave me the name of the company that made the ionizer before it was sold. It is noteworthy that some 30-years later, a company by that name still makes electrical devices with health implications according to their product catalogue.

Moreover, the reason why Walter's casual allusion to ionizing even caught my attention, was because of something I read earlier in The Body Electric. You will recall Cynthia Illingworth's discovery of regenerating fingertips in children under 11 years old (see pages 113 – 114). Well, she also observed that when the stump of an injured finger is not sewn over, it soon produces a negative electrical charge. That state seems to continue throughout the healing process. Becker also made similar observations in his work with salamander injuries.[1] The definition of *Ion* is a positive, or negative, electrical charge; *thus, where there is healing—there is ionization . . .*

---

[1] Becker, R., & Seldon, G., The Body Electric pp. 155 – 156, Chp. 4

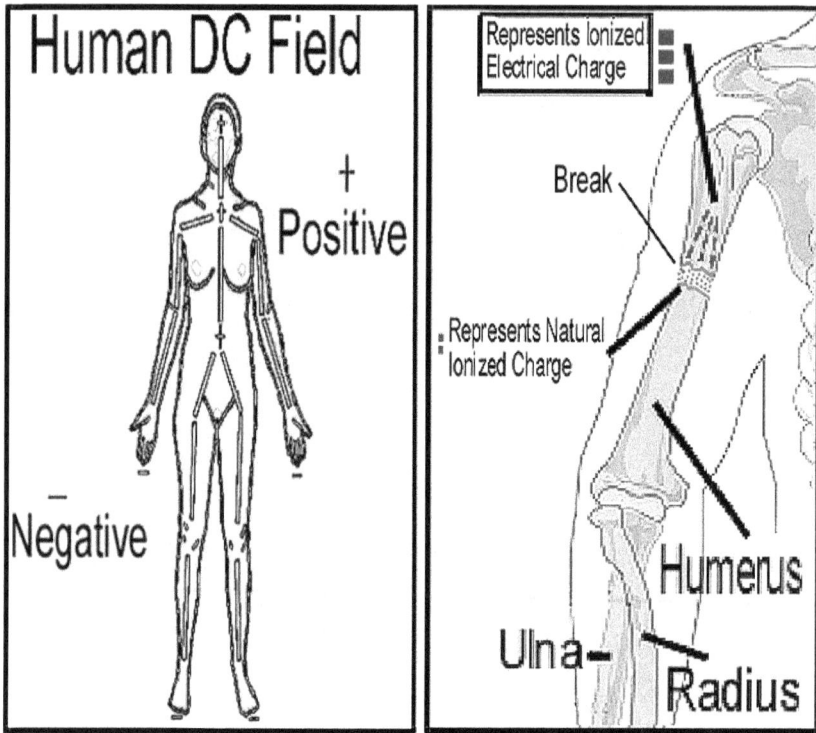

Human DC Field

+
Positive

−
Negative

Represents Ionized Electrical Charge

Break

Represents Natural Ionized Charge

Humerus

Ulna—
Radius

In actual point of fact, a hundred years ago, dentists on both sides of the Atlantic were extolling the benefits of <u>Ionic Medicine</u>! Researchers have charted the body's naturally flowing fields of positively and negatively charged electricity. In the case of injury, it appears that it is the negative charge which stimulates the healing process. Hence, one can surmise that the ionization device Walter used, *in a sense*, created a kind of natural healing environment on steroids (see diagram). After injury, the body soon produced its own natural negative charge at the site. Walter was then supplying the body with even more of that energy by creating a constant negative ionic field over the area. Illingworth found that it commonly took a young child three-months to regenerate a fingertip naturally. One only wonders how long it would take with the aid of a negatively charged electrical field?[2]

---

[2] Sturridge, E., Dental Electro-therapeutics pp. iii – iv & Levin, M., Current and potential applications of bioelectromagnetics in medicine ISSEEM Journal Vol. 4, No. 1, 1993 pp. 77 – 87

As for why ionic medicine was not mainstreamed (see page 44). Walter discusses accelerated healing on page 121. This all shared, if this chapter has been too antidotal for you, allow me to leave you with this empirically-based statement of substantiation by Dr. Michael Levin: "*Basically, the rate of bone growth and increase of mechanical integrity of knitted fractures can be accelerated noninvasively by placing a coil around the area, and creating a milliTesla AC or squarewave magnetic field by putting current through the coil. A portable version of this device, most often used for fractures that are not healing by themselves, is used in hospitals right now. There are also cases of applied electric fields being used to enhance wound healing (Carley and Wainapel, 1985). Applications are likewise being developed for treatment of ligament damage, osteoporosis, chronic skin ulcers, and tendenitis (Bassett, 1993).*" **THANK YOU WALTER!**

Life &
Electromagnetic
Energy

Some of you may be struggling with the idea of a symbiosis existing between the body and electromagnetic energy. In light of this, I felt it prudent to pen a few pages about the biological attributes of electrical energy. If you are presently wary, increasing your understanding of biology should make the science of Energetics more tenable.

In 1929, an accomplished Russian scientist named Georges Lakhovsky wrote a book entitled, <u>The Secret of Life</u>. This work explained that every biological cell has the properties of resistance, capacitance and inductance. Now what's so interesting about his disclosure is that resistance, capacitance and inductance are qualities commonly associated with electrical components. Georges Lakhovsky writes:

> " *Every living cell is essentially dependent on its nucleus which is the center of oscillations and gives off radiations . . . These nuclei are . . . actual electric circuits endowed with self-*

inductance and capacity and consequently capable of oscillating. These circuits oscillate according to a range of wavelengths whose magnitude depends essentially on the values of spirals and capacities. The waves given off are thus of electromagnetic origin . . . and are also of very high frequency and give off radiations of various frequency . . ."[1]

This was not all that Lakhovsky disclosed—he also discovered a way to kill cancer cells. His approach was to neutralize cancer cells through the use of radio wave energy. In short, after observing that cancerous cells and healthy cells have different frequencies of oscillation (movement back and

---

[1] Lakhovsky, G., <u>Secret of Life: Cosmic Rays and Radiations of Living</u> pp. 75 – 77 & Lakhovsky, G., <u>Curing Cancer with Ultra Radio Frequencies</u> & Lynes, B., <u>Cancer Solutions: Rife, Energy Medicine and Medical Politics</u> p. 50 & <u>The Granada Forum: Suppressed Medical Discovery</u> (DVD)
Lakhovsky would later state: *"Each cell is capable of being the centre of oscillations of very high frequency giving off invisible radiations belonging to a gamut close to that associated with light."*

forth) he attempted to amplify the oscillating wave frequency of the cells that were healthy, and what he found was amazing!

Amplifying the oscillations of the healthy cells literally overwhelmed the oscillatory energy of the cancer cells; eventually, causing the weaker frequency producing cancer cells to die off. Incredibly, Lakhovsky would reduce illness to nothing more than a conflict between the energy emitted from the oscillatory frequency of a healthy cell and that emitted by a diseased cell.[2]

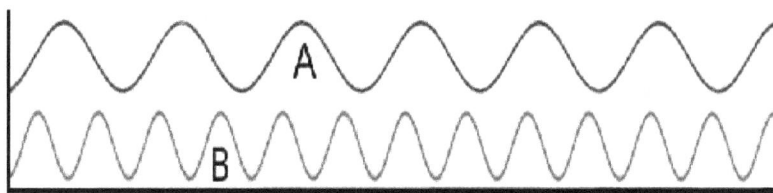

This is an example of two different cells' oscillatory wave frequencies. If the healthy cell is oscillating at the top frequency (A), that's the frequency to be amplified over the cancerous cell frequency (B) to destroy a cancer cell according to Lakhovsky.

---

[2] Lakhovsky, G., Secret of Life: Cosmic Rays and Radiations of Living Ch. VI, X & Lynes, B., Cancer Solutions: Rife, Energy Medicine and Medical Politics pp. 50 - 51

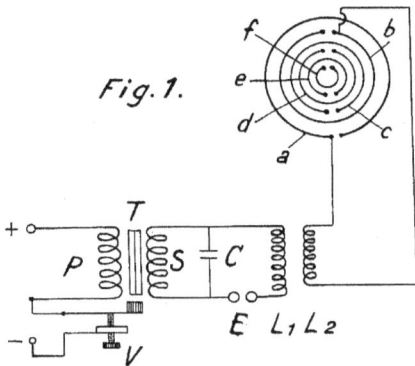

June 12, 1934.　　　G. LAKHOVSKY　　　1,962,565

APPARATUS WITH CIRCUITS OSCILLATING UNDER MULTIPLE WAVE LENGTHS

Filed Nov. 13, 1931

Fig. 1.

Fig. 2.

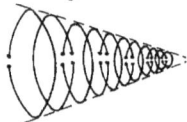

Fig. 3.

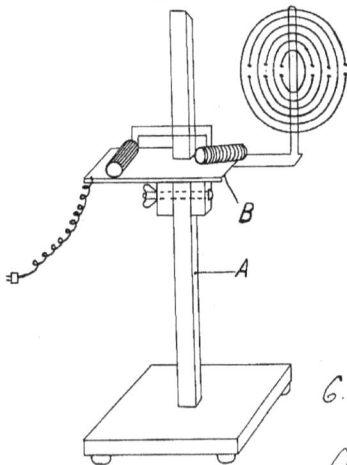

G. Lakhovsky
INVENTOR

By: Marks & Clerk
ATTYS

U.S. Patent for Lakhovsky's Multiple Wave Oscillator

About 60 years ago, another Russian scientist shared some important findings from his research with electromagnetic energy. In his studies of plants and their structures, A. M. Sinyukhin discovered that electrical energy is crucial to the healing process. Sinyukhin found that when a plant looses a limb, it generates an electrical current over the damaged area until the plant is healed. Furthermore, when he added a small electrical stimulus to a damaged plant—its healing process was accelerated over that of a damaged plant that did not receive any outside electrical stimulus. *Just one more thing to make you go—Hmmm . . .*

Coming to the 21st century, Dr. Len Horowitz makes some rather fascinating disclosures about the symbiotic relationship that exists between electromagnetic energy and human life. Briefly, everything is made up of atoms. The atom represents the smallest known division of a chemical element. All atoms are made up of three subatomic particles: they are protons, neutrons and electrons.

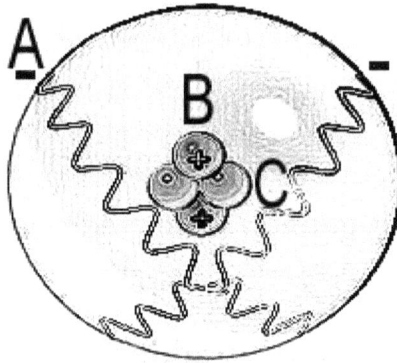

Electrons (A) are particles that have a negative electrical charge which orbit around the nucleus (in the body) of the atom. Protons (B) are much bigger and have the opposite (or positive) charge. And Neutrons (C) are the same size as protons but they have no electrical charge.

According to Horowitz, without the electro-magnetically charged protons and electrons—atoms cannot exist. ***This is the reason why biologists tell us electromagnetic energy and water are the true keys of life!***[3]

---

[3] Johnson, R., Atomic Structure & Nardo, D., Atoms
Actually, it is the unique number combination of these charged protons and electrons—which determines the

Turning to human physiology, we are constantly told that our bodies are about 70% water and that water's most important functions are to keep us hydrated and quench our thirst. In the most rudimentary sense this is correct; yet, there is a great deal more going on.[4] In addition, we are also told that the function of our DNA molecules is to house our genes, which determine such things as our height, skin color, eye color, and so forth. Yet, once more, this is only a very small part of the story.

What Dr. Len Horowitz's discloses in his <u>DNA: Pirates of the Sacred Spiral</u>, is that the principle function of DNA is to receive and transmit electromagnetic and sound wave energy! Though seemingly absurd upon first blush, this is not that radical once stopping to reflect upon the earlier

character of the atom: i.e., hydrogen, oxygen, helium, etc. Molecules are formed by combinations of similar atoms.

[4] Clayman, C., <u>The Human Body: An Illustrated Guide to its Structure, Functions, and Disorders</u> p. 175 & Heymsfield, S., & Lohman, T., & Wang, Z., & Going, S., <u>Human Body Composition</u> pp. 35 - 46

oscillatory wave findings of Georges Lakhovsky.

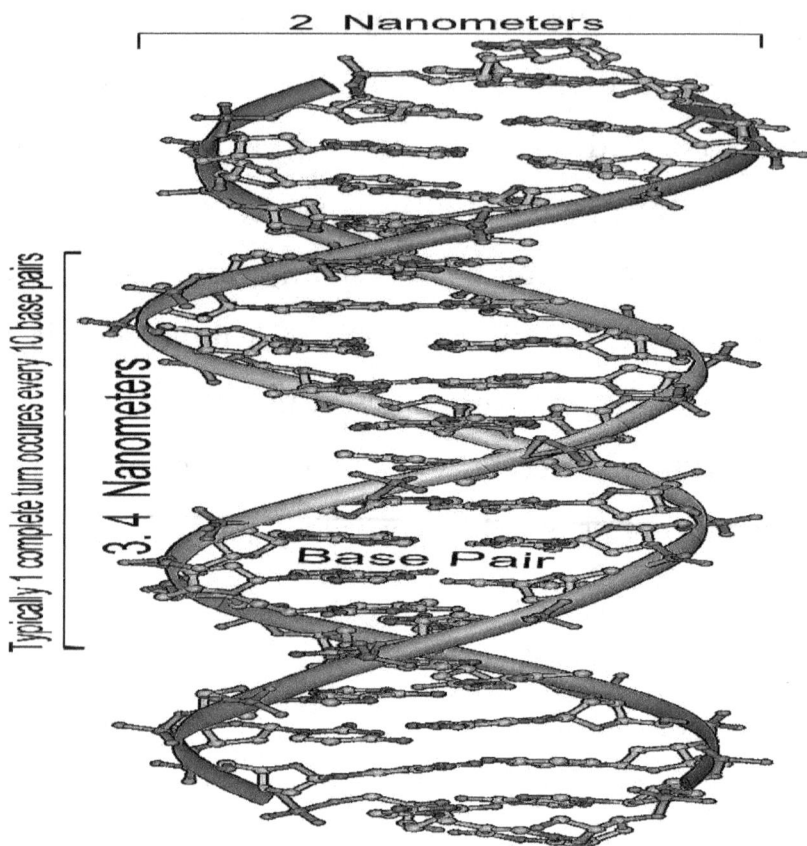

Double Helix of Deoxyribonucleic Acid (DNA)

Horowitz goes on to reveal that less than 3% of our DNA is needed to determine our entire anatomical constitution. Thus, <u>the function of the other 97% of our DNA is actually devoted to receiving and/or transmitting electromagnetic energy.</u> The reason why hydration is so essential is to facilitate that energy conduction! You see, salt water encases and supports each DNA strand. When the amount of water is insufficient, we eventually die because our DNA is unable to continue transmitting electro-magnetic energy throughout the body's cells.

Despite seeming too incredible to believe, leading scientists validate Horowitz's pronouncements. For instance, researchers in acoustic medicine explain that the sound frequency 528 (*Mi* on the music scale) is known to help repair damaged DNA. It should be noted that *Mi* literally means "MI-Ra-Gestorum" or "Miracle" in Latin. The noted biochemist Dr. Lee Lorenzen states: *"The 528 frequency is well known to scientists working on DNA repair."* Further here, Russian researchers have found that the acoustical frequencies of language itself can influence and alter human DNA![5]

---

[5] Calladine, C., & Drew, H., Understanding DNA: The Molecule & How IT Works p. 8, 13 & Horowitz, L., DNA:

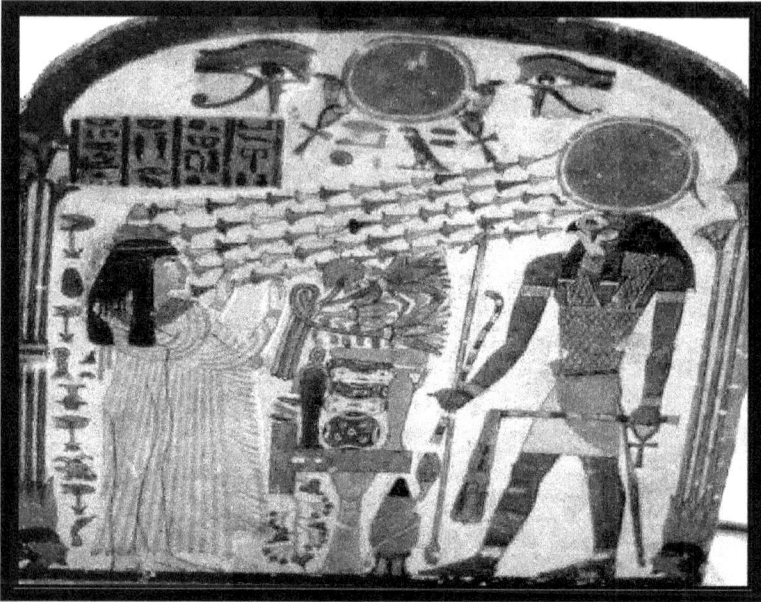

Concept of receiving invisible energy c. 1400 BCE[6]

Continuing on, the helical formation of DNA (or *Sacred Spiral* as its called by Dr. Horowitz) has long been held by scientists to actually be an electrical energy intensifying form. As a matter of fact, the

Pirates of the Sacred Spiral (DVD) & Horowitz, L., & Puleo, J., Healing Codes for the Biological Apocalypse p. 40 & Horowitz, L., & Barber, J., Ancient Healing Codes Revealed in Bible (net) & Fosar, G., & Bludorf, F., Vernetzte Intelligenz & Goldman, J., Holy Harmony (CD)
[6] Worthy, R.L., About Black Hair pp. 29 - 37
Activated-melaninized peoples' absorption and conversion of sunlight into vitamin D is one prime example of this. It is clear that the Egyptians considered the Sun to be the greatest source of life-giving electromagnetic energy in our realm.

brilliant physicist Nikola Tesla understood this and even employed it in his heralded Tesla Coil!

During his life, Tesla would be issued more than 250 patents from 25 nations. Note this remark by Tesla in the United States Patent document for his famous electromagnetic coil:

> *"I have found that in every coil there exists a certain relation between its self-induction and capacity that permits, a current of given frequency and potential to pass through it with no other opposition than that of ohmic resistance, or, in other words, as though it possessed no self-induction. This is due to the mutual relations existing between the special character of the current and the self-induction and capacity of the coil, the latter quantity being just capable of neutralizing the self-induction for that frequency . . ."*[7]

---

[7] Twenty First Century Books: <u>Coil For Electromagnets</u> (net) & (See page 127)

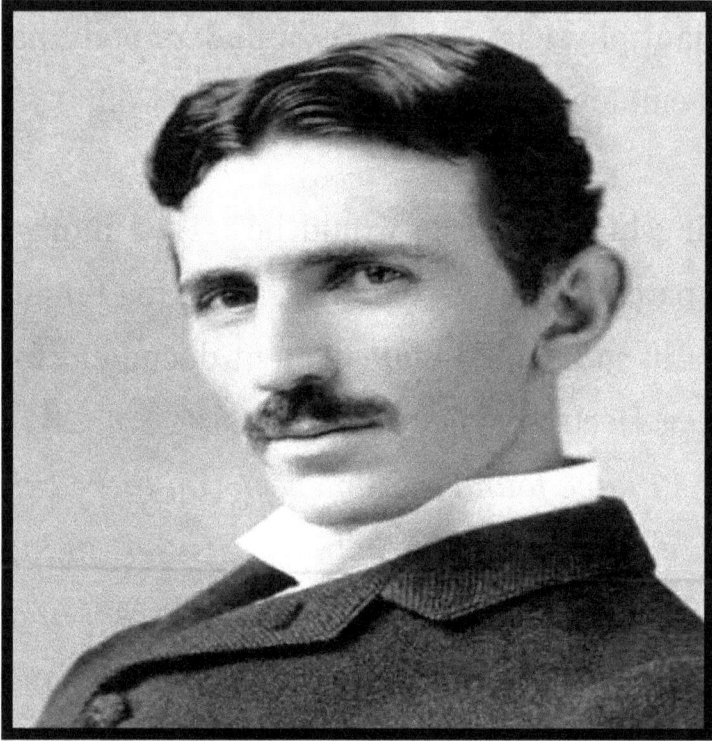

Nikola Tesla c. 1890

Say somebody—*I don't know, maybe the God of the Ages*—wanted to design something biological that was a perfect conductor of electromagnetic energy. Now let me see . . . what shape would they choose to best serve that purpose? Oh', I've got it: <u>DNA's</u>! Or, are we to conversely believe that DNA's helical design, *which speaks to perfect electrical energy conduction according to Tesla*, has absolutely no relationship to that biological function—but was just randomly selected over triangles, rectangles and squares for simple gene storage?

There is something else about the electromagnetic nature of DNA molecules that I need to share. Calladine and Drew make the point that tiny electrical charges are actually vital to the DNA strand's (see page 136) ability to maintain its helical (spiral) formation. According to our authors: *"The geometry at the core of the helix depends on subtle interactions between partial electrical charges."*[8] In other words, **no electrical energy—no DNA!**

So, after bouncing from Lakhovsky, to Sinyukhin, to Horowitz, to DNA's electrical energy intensifying structure and dependency—what have we found?

---

[8] Calladine, C., & Drew, H., Understanding DNA: The Molecule & How IT Works pp. 25 - 38
In passing, the double helix strands of DNA are found to twist in both directions—some right to left and others from left to right. The helical structure is not only found in DNA, it is also present in the body's RNA (Ribonucleic Acid).

ENERGETICS

Despite the popularized view that the human body is only basically composed of water and six fairly passive chemical elements—*we've not only found that every cell is electromagnetically charged—but that your body is actually orchestrating symphonies of synchronistic electrical operations continuously! Ergo, your body's problem isn't interacting with its electromagnetic energy—the problem begins the moment that interaction stops!*

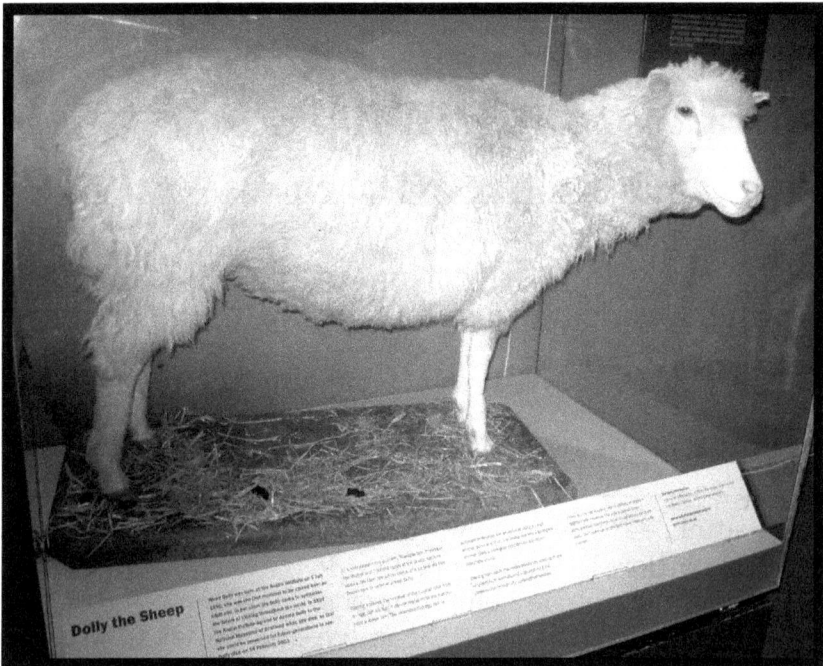

Dolly the Sheep

But even with all of this, nothing could be more illuminating about electromagnetic energy's role in life than the narrative of Dolly the Sheep! Here are the remains of Dolly, which are kept in the Museum of Scotland. Dolly was the world's first, *publicly acknowledged*, mammal to be cloned in a laboratory. Born in 1996, Dolly was created by taking the DNA of an adult sheep and scientifically inserting it into an unfertilized egg that had previously had its nucleus removed. After that, the next step was to induce cell division to start the life process by stimulating the egg with, *you guessed it*, **electromagnetic energy!**[9] Enough said.

Finally here, insomuch as the issue of cloning raises a myriad of philosophical and spiritual questions about life, allow me to leave you with this statement by Lakhovsky as it relates to electromagnetic energy and the concept of the soul:

---

[9] Williams, N., <u>Death of Dolly marks cloning milestone</u> Current Biology Vol. 13, No. 6 Mar. 2003 pp. 209 - 210

"Let us observe the fact, clearly . . . that dead plants and animals do not give any evidence of detectable radio-activity, for it appears that natural radiation is essential . . . for the maintenance of life . . . These observations, in addition to experiments on the human subject, have enabled Nodon to come to the following conclusion: 'It appears from the recorded facts that vital cells of the human body emit electrons generated by an actual radio-activity whose intensity would seem to be much more considerable than that observed in insects and plants. The fact that there should be a certain emission of energy in living beings, or a remission implying a previous activity, can hardly be doubted."[10]

---

[10] Lakhovsky, G., <u>Secret of Life: Cosmic Rays and Radiations of Living</u> pp. 80 - 81 & Horowitz, L., <u>DNA: Pirates of the Sacred Spiral</u> (DVD)
Spiritualists, Egyptologists, and those familiar with the ancient concepts of the Ba and Ka, can not help but be stimulated to intellectualization here . . .

Electromagnetic Energy & Health in History

ENERGETICS

According to Rameses II —

"The past is never dead, not even past . . ."

D espite Bob Beck's important contribution to Energetics in this age, to his great credit, he possessed enough character to explain that he was not the creator of this science, but rather, <u>a tool in its re-emergence</u>. As previously stated, energy therapy dates back at least to the time of Tesla in America. However, in actual point of fact, mankind has been treating illness with electromagnetic energy from the early dynasties of the ancient Egyptians! Thus, allow me to take a moment to share some examples of the utilization of electrical energy by healers throughout the ages . . .

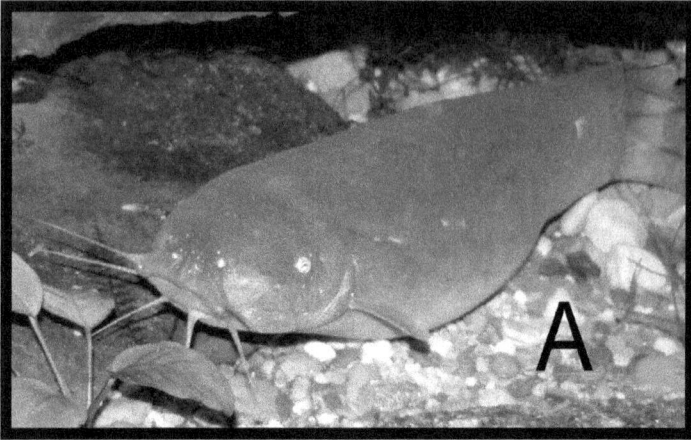

Image A is of a Nile Malapterurus electricus (a cat fish which produces an electrical charge). Stetter points out that ancient artifacts dating to c. 2500 BCE illustrate Egyptian doctors using these fish to treat their patients. Image B is of a Nile Torpedo marmorata (electric ray). The electrical current from this fish is recorded as being used to treat gout by the ancient Egyptians.EN (Endnote)

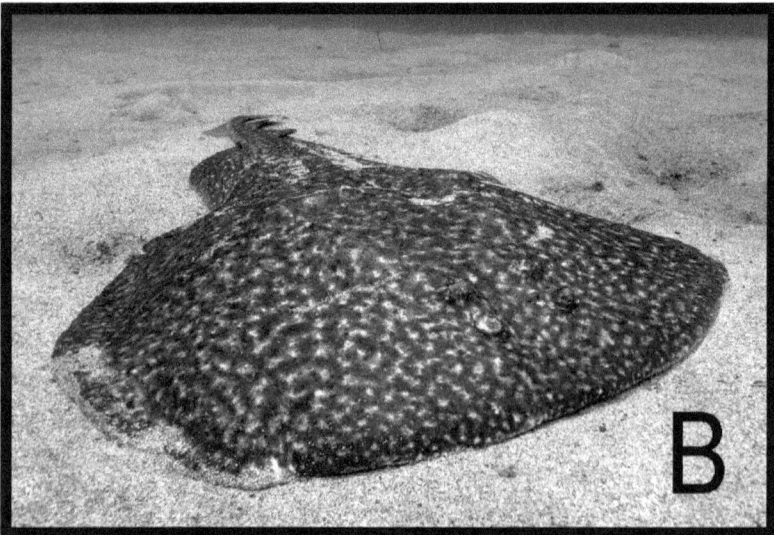

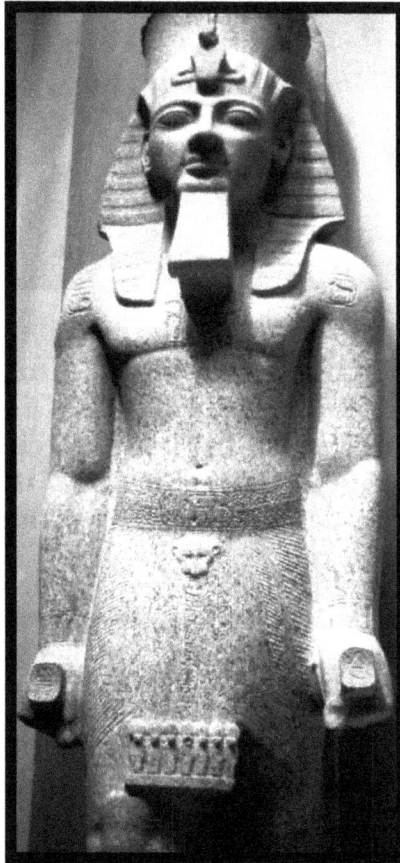

Egypt's Rameses II c. 1250 BCE

This is a statue of Rameses II. As you can see, he's firmly gripping two objects in his hands. The ancient Egyptians referred to these items as the **Wands of Horus.** Commemorated down through the ages, these devices were associated with good health for those holding them. With Konig and Wilhelm's discovery of the Baghdad battery, the discovery of many <u>electroplated</u> artifacts in Egypt's tombs, and a good deal of periphery evidence—there is reason to believe that the Wands of Horus were the world's first blood electrifying devices!EN

149

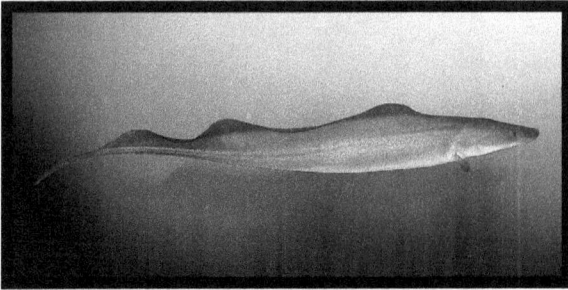

According to Brennan, the ancient Mesopotamians used electric fish to treat pain (a similar concept to that of the modern TENS machine). This is a Gymnarchus niloticus. In that electric fish were not native to the Tigris or Euphrates, it is one of the electric fish that Mesopotamian doctors may well have imported from Egypt.[EN]

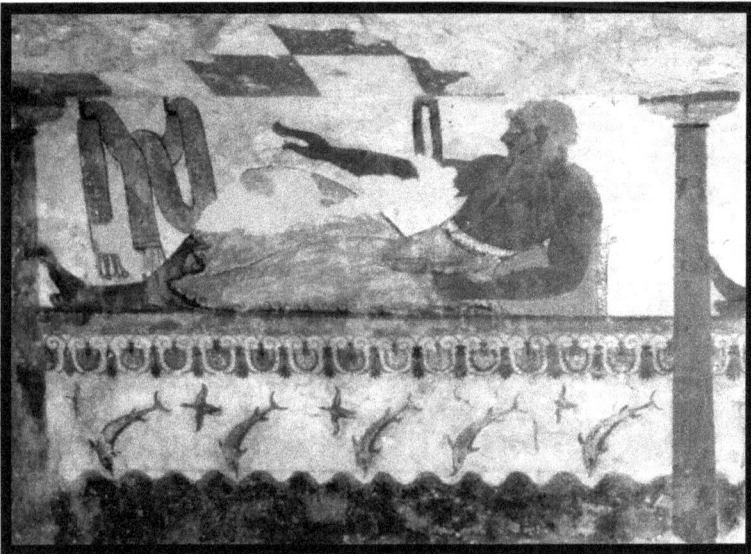

This fresco was found in the ancient Etruscan tomb of Lionus c. 600 BCE. Pliny recorded the fact that the Etruscans (founders of Rome) actually used electric fish to treat pain for gout and headache.[EN]

This is an artistic rendering of a 2nd century bas relief of the Roman Emperor Marcus Aurelius. The standing soldier has an oblong object in his hand that's being exchanged with the emperor. It must be noted that some historians have made associations between this item and the earlier Wands of Horus of the ancient Egyptians.

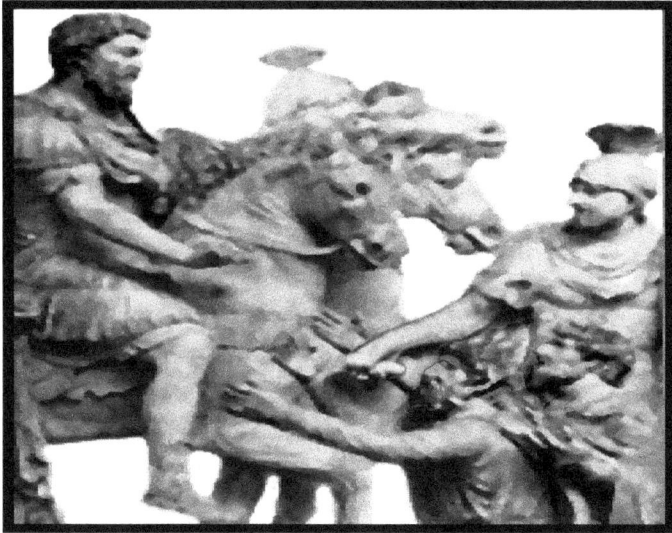

With the fall of Rome (c. 500 CE) knowledge and discovery essentially came to an end in Europe. Advancement in electrical knowledge was basically suspended until the 17th century. By the 18th century, interest in the possible health benefits of electromagnetic energy had once more taken hold. For instance, by 1750 the Scots had discovered that when a plant received electrical stimulation it grew faster than plants that did not. However, this was an unbefitting period for energy therapy. Insomuch as Europe's doctors did not associate microbes in the blood with illness—those who were using electromagnetic energy were not trying to utilize it against microorganisms. What's more, much of their early experimentation centered on pain relief. However, using Europe's unsophisticated 18th and 19th century electrical devices to treat pain, could easily produce more of it than you were originally trying to eliminate; and in fact, that is what's reported! Nevertheless, a field of medicine known as <u>Electrotherapeutics</u> would eventually take shape in Europe. In 1918, Maver wrote: *"Therapeutic electricity is used as a stimulate by its action on the nervous system and for carrying substances through the skin into the body electro-chemically. It is very useful in the hands of expert physicians but like any powerful agent, in the hands of a layman, is harmful and dangerous."*[EN]

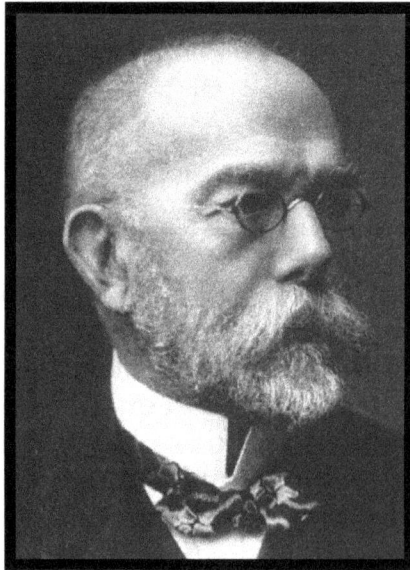

This is Robert Koch. In the 1890s he was able to verify the relationship between specific microbes and specific diseases. Today, he's seen as a pivotal figure in the area of microbiology.

By the beginning of the 20th century, advancements in Electrotherapeutics were occurring. Scientists had begun to associate microorganisms with illness. No less important, Nikola Tesla's genius and work with high frequency electrical fields made it possible to create devices that were safer and unthinkable just years earlier! This period eventually set the stage for the era of Georges Lakhovsky, Royal Rife and many Europeans in energy medicine.

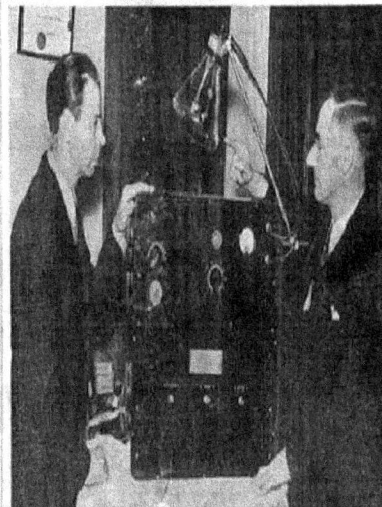

San Diego Evening Tribune May 6, 1938

During the decade of the 1920s, Royal Rife would develop two amazing inventions: first, he invented a very sophisticated electromagnetic wavelength frequency instrument, which could be calibrated to precise frequencies; and second, he produced a microscope that was capable of 17,000 magnification (or 8 times better than existing microscopes). Rife is recorded as being the first human to actually see a virus. After a conference attended by hundreds of doctors, the LA Times would describe Rife's invention as, *"The World's most Powerful Microscope!"*

In brief, Rife discovered how to destroy harmful viruses by employing the resonance principle through radio waves. In the decades leading up to his death, he would continue to make improvements to his frequency instrument and microscope. Rife would also painstakingly chart the M.O.R. (Mortal Oscillatory Rate) of many viruses.

Many cancer patients are reported as being successfully treated with Rife's machine; yet, he had, and still has, many detractors. Rife described his therapeutic procedures thus:

> *"With the frequency instrument, no tissue is destroyed, no pain is felt, no noise is audible, and no sensation is noticed. A tube lights up and 3 minutes later the treatment is complete. The virus or bacteria is destroyed and the body then recovers itself naturally from the toxic effect of the virus or bacteria . . . The first clinical work on cancer was completed under the supervision of Milbank Johnson, M.D. which was set up under a Special Medical Research Committee of the*

*University of Southern California. 16 cases were treated at the clinic for many types of malignancy. After 3 months, 14 of these so called hopeless cases were signed off as clinically cured by the staff of five medical doctors and Dr. Alvin G. Foord, M.D. Pathologist for the group . . ."*EN

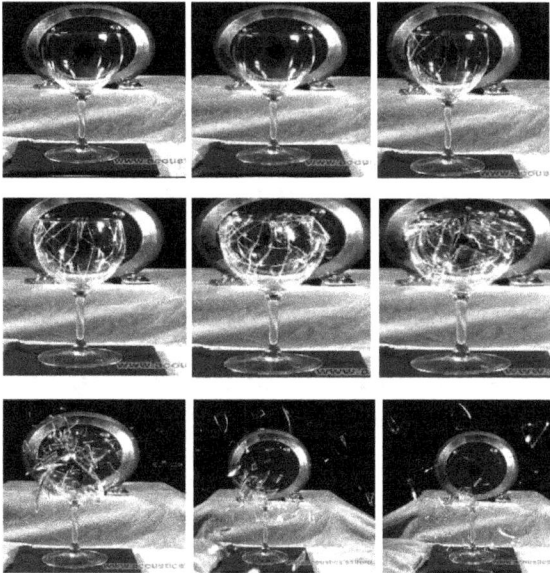

A final point here about the Rife controversy: an example of the principle of resonance is clearly demonstrated above with this crystal glass. When the proper sound wave energy is directed at the glass and amplified beyond its safe resonance (vibratory) point for a sufficient period of time—the vibration ultimately causes the glass to shake apart (or shatter). Believe it or not, modern researchers have successfully applied this resonance principle against microorganisms—essentially exploding them! In the words of Blake: *"What is now proved, was only once imagined . . ."*EN

155

ENERGETICS

If the truth is to be told, Americans were not the only practitioners of electromagnetic therapeutics during the past century:

Niels Finsen was a Danish/Icelandic physician who won the Nobel Prize in Medicine in 1903, for his work with ultraviolet light energy and microbes. What he discovered was that microorganisms are highly susceptible to energy from ultraviolet light!

By the 1920s, there appear to have been a significant number of British physicians and dentists touting electric medicine; prescribing it for many illnesses!

In the 1930s, the Chinese had begun to combine electricity with acupuncture treatment!

The 40s would usher in the therapeutic application of ultra sound energy technology!

The fact is that the Russians, Germans and French were all investigating electrotherapeutics. Indeed, in <u>Bioelectromagnetic Medicine</u>, Dr. Rosch explains that from the 1920s onward, many scientists wrote well-regarded textbooks about the therapeutic promise of electromagnetic energy!

We even find Energetics being used to treat cancer (<u>underground</u>) around the world for decades!

To close out the century back in America, we've already discussed the important contributions of Kaali, Lyman, and Schwolsky. On the ensuing page we have Kaali and Schwolsky's Patent 5,188,738. The text at the bottom is lines 27 – 40 of the <u>Practical Uses of Invention</u> section of the patent.

United States Patent [19]   US005188738A

Kaali et al.   [11] Patent Number: 5,188,738
                                [45] Date of Patent: * Feb. 23, 1993

[54] ALTERNATING CURRENT SUPPLIED
ELECTRICALLY CONDUCTIVE METHOD
AND SYSTEM FOR TREATMENT OF
BLOOD AND/OR OTHER BODY FLUIDS
AND/OR SYNTHETIC FLUIDS WITH
ELECTRIC FORCES

[76] Inventors: Steven Kaali, 88 Ashford Ave.,
Dobbs Ferry, N.Y. 10522; Peter M.
Schwolsky, 4101 Cathedral Ave.,
NW., Washington, D.C. 20016

[*] Notice: The portion of the term of this patent
subsequent to Aug. 18, 2009 has been
disclaimed.

[21] Appl. No.: 615,437

[22] Filed: Nov. 16, 1990

Related U.S. Application Data

[63] Continuation-in-part of Ser. No. 562,721, Aug. 6, 1990,
abandoned.

[51] Int. Cl.⁵ 301D 35/06; A61K 41/00
[52] U.S. Cl. .... 210/748; 128/419 R;
128/421; 128/783; 128/784; 204/131; 204/164;
204/186; 204/302; 210/243; 422/22; 422/44;
604/4
[58] Field of Search 210/243, 748, 764;
128/419 R, 421, 783, 784; 604/4; 422/22, 44;
204/131, 164, 186, 242, 275, 302, 305

[56]   References Cited
U.S. PATENT DOCUMENTS

592,735	10/1897	Jones	204/242
672,231	4/1901	Lacomme	204/275
2,490,730	12/1949	Dubilier	204/305
3,692,648	9/1972	Matloff et al.	204/129
3,753,886	8/1973	Myers	204/186
3,878,564	4/1975	Yao et al.	210/648
3,965,008	6/1976	Dawson	422/22
3,994,799	11/1976	Yao et al.	210/321.64
4,473,449	9/1984	Michaels et al.	204/101
4,616,640	10/1986	Kaali et al.	128/130
4,770,167	9/1988	Kaali et al.	128/788
4,932,421	6/1990	Kaali et al.	128/831
5,049,252	9/1991	Murrell	210/243
5,058,065	10/1991	Slovak	128/783
5,133,932	7/1992	Gunn et al.	210/748

FOREIGN PATENT DOCUMENTS

995848 7/1983 U.S.S.R. 210/243

OTHER PUBLICATIONS

Proceedings of the Society for Experimental Biology &
Medicine, vol. 1, (1979), pp. 204–209, "Inactivation of
Herpes Simples Virus with Methylene Blue, Light and
Electricity"—Mitchell R. Swartz et al.
Journal of the Clinical Investigation published by the
American Society for Clinical Investigations, Inc., vol.
65, Feb. 1980, pp. 432–438—"Mechanisms of Photody-
namic Inactivation of Herpes Simplex Viruses"
—Lowell E. Schnipper et al.
Journal of Clinical Microbiology, vol. 17, No. 2, Feb.
1983, pp. 374–376, "Photodynamic Inactivation of
Pseudorabier Virus with Methylene Blue Dye, Light
and Electricity"—Janine A. Badyisk et al.

Primary Examiner—Robert A. Dawson
Assistant Examiner—Sun Uk Kim
Attorney, Agent, or Firm—Charles W. Helzer

[57]   ABSTRACT

A new alternating current process and system for treatment of blood and/or other body fluids and/or synthetic fluids from a donor to a recipient or storage receptacle or in a recycling system using novel electrically conductive treatment vessels for treating blood
and/or other body fluids and/or synthetic fluids with
electric field forces of appropriate electric field strength
to provide electric current flow through the blood or
other body fluids at a magnitude that is biologically
compatible but is sufficient to render the bacteria, virus,
parasites and/or fungus ineffective to infect or affect
normally healthy cells while maintaining the biological
usefulness of the blood or other fluids. For this purpose
low voltage alternating current electric potentials are
applied to the treatment vessel which are of the order of
from about 0.2 to 12 volts and produce current flow
densities in the blood or other fluids of from one microampere per square millimeter of electrode area exposed
to the fluid being treated to about two milliamperes per
square millimeter.

31 Claims, 6 Drawing Sheets

through a portion of the length of the vessel, and means
for applying low voltage alternating current non-bio-
logically damaging electric potentials to the electrically
conductive electrode segments whereby electrical field
forces are produced between the electrically conductive electrode segments that induce biologically compatible current flow through the blood and/or other
fluids contained in or flowing through the vessel so as to
attenuate bacteria, virus, parasites and/or fungus contained in the blood and/or other fluids by the action of
the electric current flow therethrough to thereby render the bacteria, virus, parasites and/or fungus ineffective while not impairing and maintaining the biological
usefulness of the fluids.

ENERGETICS

EXPERIMENTAL IN VIVO BLOOD VIRUS, MICROBE, FUNGI, AND PARASITE
ELIMINATION DEVICE
Revision March 16, 1996 Copyright © 1993/1996 Robert C. Beck

Note: These data are for informational, instructional, and research purposes only and are not to be construed as medical advice.
Consult your licensed medical practitioner.

CHANGES since previous editions: Pulse Repetition Rate from 0.67 to ~4 Hz. (Not critical). C 2 from 1 to 0.22μF. Voltage from 36 to 27V. Treatment time increased to 2 hours daily for 21 to 30 days. Improved electrode design and single wrist electrode placement. SW 2 added to extend battery life. There are NO "errors" in this schematic. Hundreds have been constructed successfully when duplicated exactly without user attempted "improvements".

As heretofore mentioned, this is the paradigm altering microorganism elimination device of Bob Beck. __The significance of his contribution to the area of blood electrification and electromagnetic pulsing is that he produced instruments which make it possible for anyone to safely perform these procedures in vivo as opposed to in vitro.__ Thus, if the Sun shines where you live, you can investigate this! We are all greatly indebted to this physicist for having the moral fiber to use his knowledge in low-level electrical fields for good and not for ill.[EN]

In winding up, there is no doubt as to the linkage between electrical energy and health. We have discussed the electromagnetic changes that occur in plants and humans when a limb is damaged. No less compelling, <u>European researchers even disclose the fact that our antibodies actually utilize electrical energy to destroy invading organisms</u>! As a matter of fact, even when the heart suddenly stops—doctors don't prescribe aspirin or order filet mignon—*they immediately apply electricity to the heart: Paddles, Stand-Back, CHARGING—**<u>CLEAR!!!</u>***[1]

Since the word *health* literally means "wholeness," *illness* implies some deficit. In light of the vital role that electrical energy plays in biology, the question is rather obvious: *Why shouldn't we consider safe energy augmentation for some illness—as opposed*

---

[1] Becker, R., & Selden, G., <u>The Body Electric: Electromagnetism And The Foundation of Life</u> & <u>The Beck Protocol</u> (DVD) & <u>Bioelectric Medicine</u>
The heart and nerves cannot function without electrical energy. It should also be noted that allopaths have begun to use electromagnetic devises to treat migraine headache.

to tersely prescribing, and even mixing, side-effect producing drugs, and/or cutting to alter or remove body parts—for practically all? According to Rife:

> *"In reality, it is not the bacteria themselves that produce the disease, but the chemical constituents of these microorganisms enacting upon the unbalanced cell metabolism of the human body that in actuality produce the disease. We also believe if the metabolism of the human body is perfectly balanced or poised, it is susceptible to no disease."*[2]

It has been irrefutably established that microcurrents immobilize microorganisms.

Let me close with one final observation about electromagnetic energy and healing. Today, many

---

[2] Lynes, B., The Cancer Cure That Worked! & Lynes, B., Cancer Solutions: Rife, Energy Medicine and Medical Politics
On the other hand, I have met a countless number of sick people who routinely take between 20 and 30 pills a day, month after month, year after year—*only to remain sick . . .*

health associations consider the Ophiuchus (pronounced OFF-ee-YOO-kuss) to be the universal symbol of health. In the Western medical tradition, the Ophiuchus is heralded as the 13th zodiacal sign ("The Serpent Bearer"). The Serpent Bearer is seen as a man with who was granted great medical knowledge by the gods. Using this knowledge wisely, he was eventually placed in the heavens. The Greeks would eventually refer to him as Asclepius.

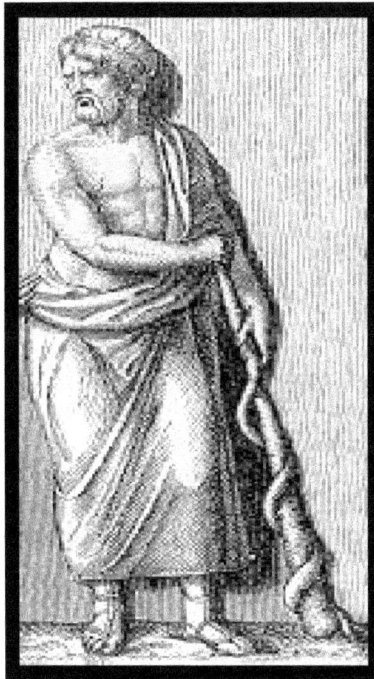

Western writers also tell us he used a stick to control worms when conducting some medical treatments; hence, their explanation for the serpent and staff imagery.

The Serpent Bearer

In passing, a Western connection between the Ophiuchus and healing has also been made because of the snake's ability to shed its skin: some ancient writers considering this unique faculty to represent an understanding of life regeneration.[3]

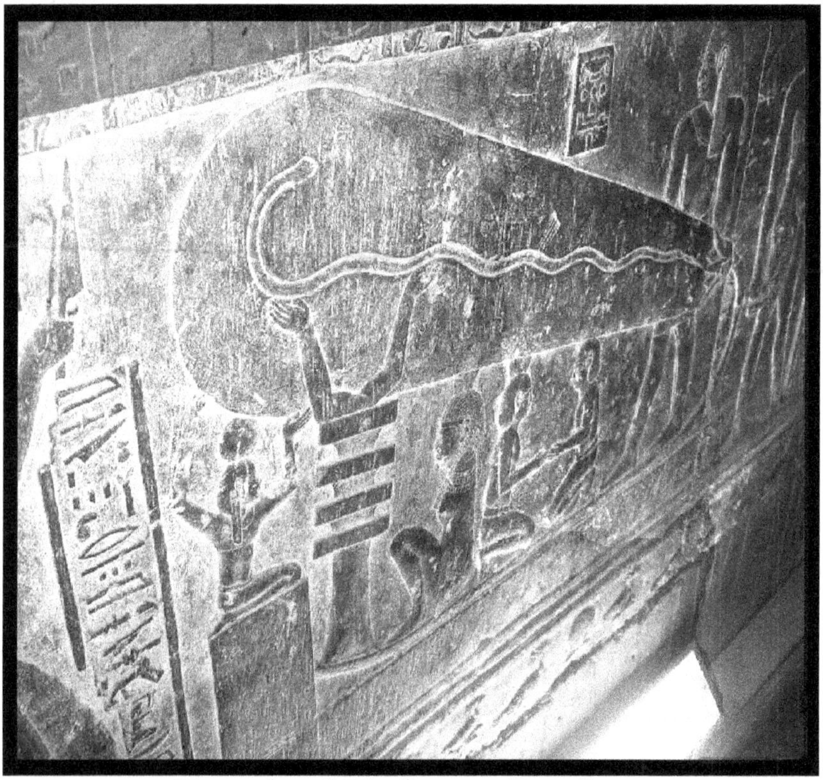

Temple of Hathor at Dendera

[3] Heifetz, M., & Tirion, W., A Walk through the Southern Sky pp. 87 - 88 & Blayney, K., The Caduceus vs the Staff of Asclepius (net) & Michon, G., Scientific Symbols and Icons: The rod of Aesculapius (net)

However, in truth, this symbol is much older than the Greeks. For example, amongst the earlier African doctors of ancient Egypt, the Ophiuchus possessed profound meaning. For starters, the staff and serpent imagery was seen as <u>The Rod of Imhotep</u> (*Imhotep being the world's oldest empirical physician*).[4] What's more, the serpent glyph was, in fact, a designation for electromagnetic energy! Nowhere has evidence of this been more conspicuous than in the ancient Egyptian Temple of Hathor at Dendera.[5] *As is often the case—people look, but so seldom do they see . . .*

---

[4] The later Greek God of Medicine, Asclepius, is an allusion to Imhotep of the ancient Egyptians (see pages 4 – 9).

[5]De Lubicz, R., <u>Sacred Science: The King of Pharaonic Theocracy</u> & <u>Ancient Lives</u> (VHS) & Clark, R., <u>The Sacred Tradition in Ancient Egypt</u> & Berlitz, C., <u>The Bermuda Triangle</u> & Stetter, C., <u>The Secret Medicine of the Pharaohs</u> & Tesla, N., & Childress, D., <u>The Fantastic Inventions of Nikola Tesla</u> & Berlitz, C., <u>Atlantis: The Eighth Continent</u> & Warren, L., <u>Did Ancient Cultures know about Electricity</u>? Plim Report (net) & Electronics 101: <u>Fundamentals of Electricity</u> (net) & Tompkins, P., <u>The Magic of Obelisks</u> & Worthy, R.L., <u>YHSVH</u>

The fact that the ancients utilized electricity is well known in the academic community; indeed, the discovery of the Baghdad Battery leaves no doubt amongst academics.

Thus, for the world's first physicians, the symbol of the staff and the coiled serpent had a far deeper literal significance than the afore mentioned Greek mythology: the staff represented the spine (core) of the human body; while the serpent represented the electromagnetic energy that envelops and coils around that axis![6] *Ergo, the actual meaning of the oldest symbol for healing known to mankind is "Human Mass and Electromagnetic Energy!"*

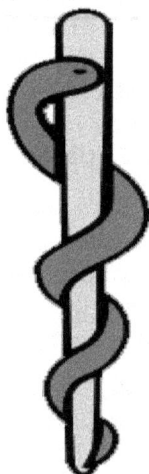

---

[6] Brugsch-Bey, H., & Seymour, H., <u>A History of Egypt Under the Pharaohs</u> p. 422
The ancient Chakra and Kundalini systems of the Western Asia are also thought to be expressions of this concept. It's also noteworthy that well into the later centuries, the serpent glyph still symbolized electricity amongst Coptic Egyptians.

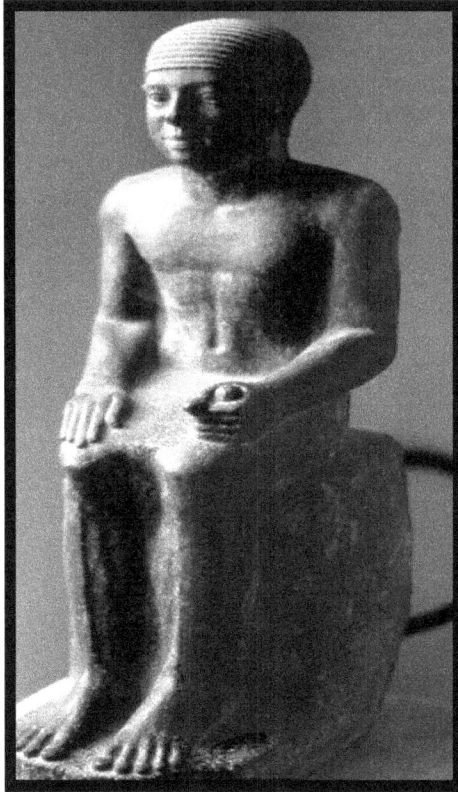

**Egyptian noble holding
One Wand of Horus c. 2000 BCE**

King Solomon and other philosophers down through the ages have explained: *"There is nothing new under the Sun!"* Whether they are right or wrong—*I suggest you begin to investigate taking back your power . . .*

165

ENERGETICS

MY FELLOW RESEARCHERS, I HAVE NO FORMAL TRAINING IN ALLOPATHIC MEDICINE. FURTHERMORE, THIS IS NOT A BOOK ABOUT TREATING ANY SPECIFIC DISEASE; E.G., HIV, BREAST CANCER, HERPES, MENINGITIS, HEPATITIS, PROSTATE CANCER, ETC. THAT SAID, I AM AN AUTODIDACTIC RESEARCHER OF ENERGETICS. THIS WORK RELATES TO A SAFE AND SCIENTIFICALLY PROVEN METHOD FOR HELPING THE BODY TO ELIMINATE THE MICROBIAL CAUSE OF THESE, AND OTHER, MALADIES. LASTLY, THE A.M.A. AND LAW OF THE LAND REQUIRE THAT THE INFORMATION IN THIS BOOK BE INTENDED FOR RESEARCH AND/OR THEORETICAL PURPOSES ONLY—AND NOT BE SEEN AS MEDICAL ADVICE . . .

166

Endnotes:

Stetter, C., The Secret Medicine of the Pharaohs pp. 107 – 108, bk-cover & Brennan, H., The Secret history of Ancient Egypt pp. 93 – 109 & Tompkins, P., The Magic of Obelisks p. 456 & Arthur C. Clarke's Mysterious World: Ancient Wisdom Vol. V (VHS) 1980 & Berlitz, C., Mysteries From Forgotten Worlds p. 24 & Maver, W., Electricity, its History and Progress, The Encyclopedia Americana; a library of Universal knowledge Vol. X, pp. 171 - 173 & Brugsch-Bey, H., & Seymour, H., A History of Egypt Under the Pharaohs p. 422 & Morris, S., Life's Solution: Inevitable Humans in a Lonely Universe pp. 182 – 185 & Brock, T., Robert Koch: A Life in Medicine and Bacteriology & Lynes, B., Cancer Solutions: Rife, Energy Medicine and Medical Politics pp. 47 – 48, 100 –103, 117 – 118 & The Rife Microscope Cancer Cure Story (net) & Bailey, D., & Wright, E., Practical Fiber Optics p. 23 & Lynes. B., The Cancer Cure That Worked pp. 34 – 36, 43 – 47, 51, 60 – 61, 72 – 73 & Essential Atlas of Physiology pp. 82 – 83 & Garratt, A., Medical Electricity & Niels Ryberg Finsen: Wikipedia (net) & Armstrong, J., The Water of life p. 25 & Dharmananda, S., ELECTRO-ACUPUNCTURE (net) & Becker, R., & Seldon, G., The Body Electric pp. 233 – 236 & Berlitz, C., Atlantis: The Eighth Continent pp. 128 - 129 & The World's Strangest UFO Stories (DVD) & Plim Report: Did Ancient Cultures know about Electricity? (net) & Electronics 101: Fundamentals of Electricity (net) & Electric Battery, The World Book Encyclopedia Vol. V, p. 2248, Vol. V, p. 2280, Vol. X, p. 435, Vol. XX, p. 446 & De Lubicz, R., Sacred Science: The King of Pharaonic Theocracy p. 114 & Iron, Metallurgy of, Universal Standard Encyclopedia Vol. XIII, p. 4436 & Van Sertima, I., Blacks in Science: ancient and modern p. 9 & Malek, J., & Forman, W., In the Shadow of the Pyramids p. 31 Daniel, G., Nubia Under the Pharaohs pp. 66 - 67 & & Budge, E.A., The Dwellers on the Nile pp. 37, 60 – 61 & The Old Kingdom and First Intermediate Period (PDF) Cleveland Museum of Art pp. 50-53 & Worthy, R.L. The Racialization of Slavery p. 95

As for why Royal Rife's discoveries were not more widely received, insomuch as they were a direct threat to the profits and control of the MIC (see pages 36 – 53) they were systematically suppressed. Over and above that, not only was Rife harassed—but two of his staunchest early supporters died mysteriously: Dr. Milbank Johnson was poisoned just hours before he was to give a public address pronouncing the promise of Rife's work; and Dr. Nemes, who was testing and affirming Rife's claims—was killed in a suspicious laboratory fire shortly thereafter. Of course, the instant reaction of many of you will be to dismiss any idea of corporate malfeasance, and chock these deaths up to sheer coincidence. However, my considered reply to you is this—*After decades of service to the wealthy of this nation, Major General Smedley Butler – U.S. Marine Corps, would in all likelihood, **beg to differ**!* In closing, Royal Rife died in 1971 from a lethal overdose of Valium given to him during, *you guessed it*, a stay in the hospital . . .

Sexual Health

WARNING—SOME GRAPHIC IMAGERY

S ex is a <u>life affirming act</u>! Despite the current push to only view sex through a Western European prism, the fact is that sex has been explored, understood and appreciated by all of humanity down through the ages; *and with no less vim or vigor I might add.* As one ancient Egyptian woman was to say to her beloved: *"Here, take my breast—they are full to overflowing, and all for you—glorious is the day of our lovemaking!"*[1]

An Egyptian love song explained-I will lie down in my house, I will lie ill, something will happen to me, and the neighbors will visit me. My lover will come too and she will shame them all, the doctors and everyone else, because she has the cure for my disease!

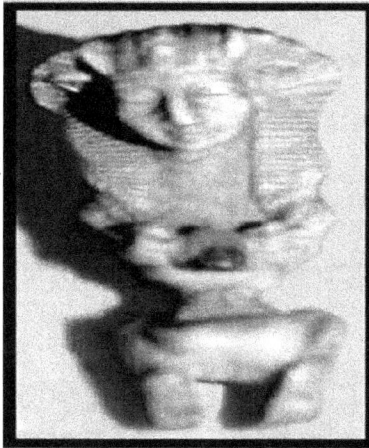

Egyptian Lovers c. 1450 BCE

---

[1] Stetter, C., <u>Secret Medicine of the Pharaohs</u> pp 85 - 89 & <u>Song of Songs</u> & Bechtel, S., & Stains, L., <u>Sex: A Man's Guide</u> p. 211 & Kaster, J., <u>Wings of the Falcon: Life and Thought of Ancient Egypt</u> p. 226
This artifact is a part of the British Museum Collection of Egyptian Antiquities.

Believe me, I have no inclination to write a treatise about sex. Yet, there are forces that want to transform this wonderful blessing into a curse; namely, *this physically and emotionally gratifying act of life (coitus) being misapplied so as to literally culminate in poor health and death.*

Before you can be deceived, you must be convinced of a lie. It doesn't matter if it is a well-conceived falsehood or one that's poorly developed. One of the most dangerous deceptions propagated today is that there's no significant sexual difference between the anus and vagina; making them interchangeable . . .

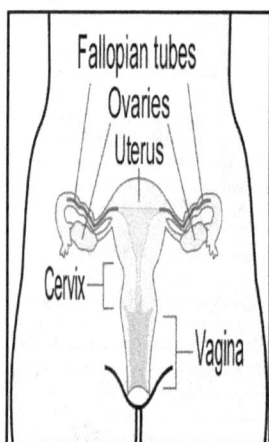
Diagram 1

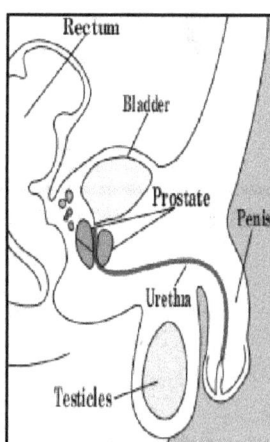
Diagram 2

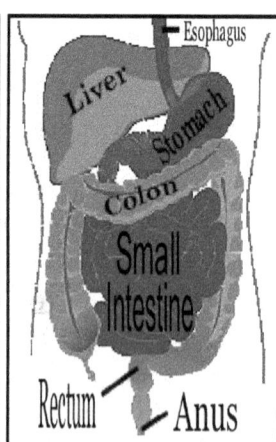
Diagram 3

The diagrams on the preceding page illustrate human anatomy. When it comes to coitus, the body has well-developed sensitive organs (genitalia) which give humans the ability to have exciting orgasms and to reproduce: they are the *vagina* of the female and the *penis* of the male. When examining diagrams 1 and 2, it is clear that the vagina and penis are organs that are literal channels of life. The uterus and vagina are the canals that eggs flow through to be fertilized by the sperm, which is inserted into the female through the male penis. This is how primates procreate; hence my use of the phrase, **life affirming act.**

On the other hand, in the case of the anus what's found is not merely different—*it is the exact opposite!* If the vagina and penis are said to be channels of life, the anus and rectum can literally be described as passageways of dissolution and death. I say this because the moment nourishment touches the tongue, the digestive process begins; if it didn't we would starve. Diagram 3 helps us to see that as food travels through the digestive tract, it soon reaches the stomach where hydrochloric acid kills many harmful microorganisms and breaks the food down even further. Typically taking a few hours, the resulting liquid first passes through the small intestine and then into the colon; this is when the nutrients are actually absorbed into the body. After that process, the body has no use for the remaining toxic matter (*feces*) so it is passed on to the rectum and ultimately evacuated out of the anus.[2]

Look, I am not trying to judge anyone's sexual orientation. Regardless of your orientation, to substitute a virulent passageway for one that is not, could prove to be a fatal mistake. According to Daily and Ehrlich:

> *"Death rates from many diseases were lowered dramatically in today's developed*

---

[2] By contrast, proteins and vitamins can even be said to pass through the life affirming passages of the penis and vagina.

nations long before antibiotics or other effective medical interventions were available . . . This was accomplished with improved nutrition, housing less available to vermin, cleaner drinking water, <u>improved isolation from human fecal contamination</u>, and soap."[3]

What these scientists are explaining is that avoiding feces was a milestone in man's pursuit of good health and longer life! Modern researchers estimate the annual worldwide loss of life and infection due to fecal contamination to be in the millions. Here are some of the common pathogenic microbes found in feces: Escherichia coli (E. coli); salmonella; candida; cryptosporidium; aeromonas; and several other harmful bateroides.

Another point that needs to be made here is that the illnesses born from these microbes are not always

---

[3] Daily, G., & Ehrlich, P., <u>DEVELOPMENT, GLOBAL CHANGE, AND EPIDEMIOLOGICAL ENVIRONMENT</u> pp. 13 - 14

immediate in their presentation. For example, this happens to be so with cholera and the disease Hepatitis A, which attacks the liver.[4]

Young people, there are powerful and influential entities on this planet who do not have your best interest at heart.[5] The purpose of the images and lies you are being force-fed is not entertainment or enlightenment; it's to keep you lost in your place. Ergo, pimping the pleasure principle was simply designed to turn healthy and sensuous beings into unhealthy viral incubators. Thus be forewarned, following the crowd may not get you where you

---

[4] Cholera: a Deadly Infection Bukisa (net) & Beckingham, R., ABC of disease of liver, pancreas and biliary system: Acute hepatitis BMJ Vol. 322 No. 7279 pp. 151–153 & Bain, V., & Ma, M., Acute Viral Hepatitis Chp. 14
It could be months before any disturbing symptoms appear.
[5] Horowitz, L., Emerging Viruses DVD & Jones, A., Endgame DVD & Horowitz, L., DNA: Pirates of the Sacred Spiral DVD
In truth, Dr. Leonard Horowitz, Daniel Eustulin, David Icke, Dr. Stanley Monteith, Dr. Michael Coffman, Jim Tucker, Alex Jones, Jeremy Wright, and Dr. Rima Laibow have all come forward to expose the "Great Culling" of the "Useless Eaters" that's been planned by the elite (see pages 189, 195 - 199).

really want to go. Indeed, when it comes to coitus—random partnering, inane, anal, and bestial sex can literally lead you into a dead end.[6]

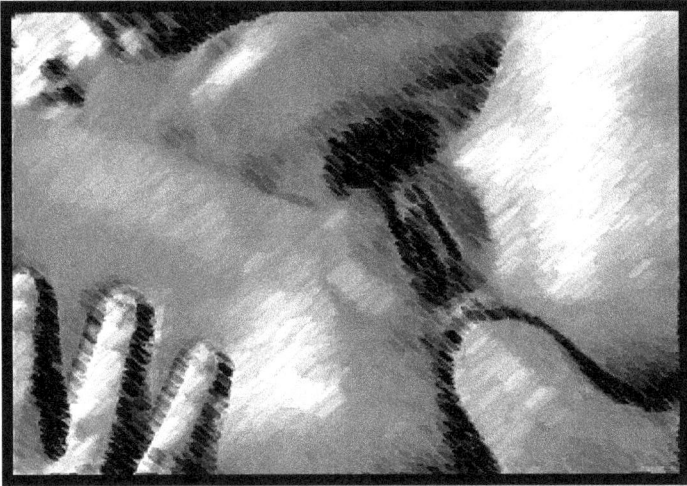

Having shared all of that, let me say this: *In light of the verified science, if you have health concerns related to your sex life (regardless of what you've read or been told elsewhere) your investigation of Energetics is well-warranted![7]*

---

[6] The reason abdominal injuries are so dangerous is because of the deadly infections that can occur from fecal microbes. Fecal microorganisms typically enter the body through the mouth or a break in the skin.

[7] The Granada Forum: Suppressed Medical Discovery (DVD) & The Beck Protocol (DVD)
Remember, microcurrents immobilize all microorganisms.

Bob C. Beck for one, *and I for another*, are witnesses to this fact. In deference here to Beck:

> *"The blood of an AIDS patient is extraordinary to look at under a microscope. What you see will just shock you. There are life forms in their blood that look like octopuses with a hundred arms, and there are things creeping around. Then we look at their blood after a few weeks [of energy therapy] and all of these things are disappearing. Their blood returns to the natural healthy state . . ."*[8]

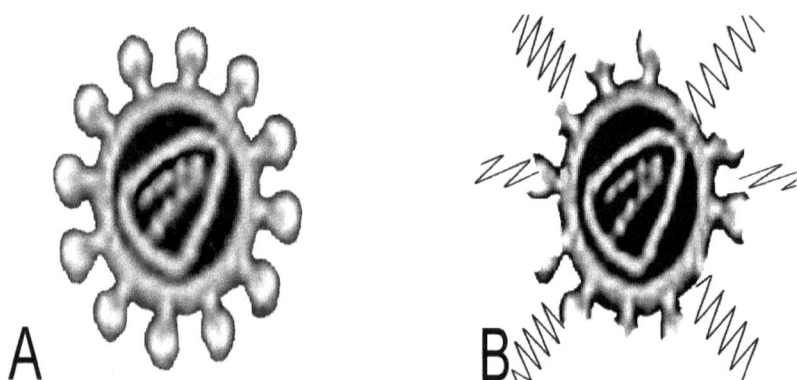

A   B

---

[8] Global Sciences Congress: THE BOB BECK INTERVIEW
Image A represents a normal pathogenic microorganism (e.g., HIV, Herpes, Epstein Bar, etc.). However, image B represents the same microorganism after energy therapy.

My Testimony

ENERGETICS

During the 70s, 80s and 90s, I was keen and blessed to travel the world. I also zigzagged across America a few times in that period. Eager to taste the fruit of many lands and regions—*I did*. As fate would have it, along the way I contracted Genital herpes (*not in Bangkok, Dar es Salaam, Paris or Amsterdam—but a few miles from my home in the U.S., and from a 'nice girl'—go figure*). Nevertheless, she had it—we did it—and I got it . . .

For twenty years I endured the episodic headaches, ulcerations and fevers that are the gifts of this disease to its carriers.[1] Not just that, there was also the matter of trying not to give it to anyone else!

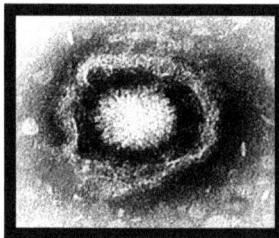

Herpesviridae

---

[1] Approximately every 10 - 12 weeks in my case.

But being healthy all my life, it took a while for me to actually accept the idea of having a virus that my body couldn't naturally fight off. Once coming to that realization, I began looking for a remedy in conventional medicine. All I found there was, *"Genital herpes is common amongst men and women in the United States"* and *"There is no cure for Genital herpes."*[2] After a time, I learned to live with it; and besides, if 50 million other Americans have Genital herpes, *what's the big deal—right?*

Well, I limped along like that for about twenty years until I saw the Strecker Memorandum (*a very important work*). Although Strecker's work focused on HIV, I found the idea of resonance being applied to healing fascinating. My study of the resonance principle introduced me to Rife's work, which shortly thereafter led me to the work of Tesla, Lakhovsky and a host of others. In the course of

---

[2] United States Centers for Disease Control and Prevention

that research, I came across the concept of blood electrification and Dr. Bob Beck. **Here was a respected physicist explaining that not only were all microorganisms controllable, but the United States Government had already patented devices which did precisely that!**

After investigating the patents and finding Beck to be spot on, I decided that twenty years was long enough to carry the herpes virus unnecessarily. No less disturbing, when news broke in 1993 that HIV could be attenuated through blood electrification, the forecast was that it would take about 15 years for the process to be perfected for humans. As if that prediction wasn't foreboding enough considering the fatal toll of AIDS annually—*it had already been 15 years from the 1993 discovery* (see page 157) *to my introduction to Beck's work*—and blood electrification wasn't, and still isn't, even on the public's radar! *I wonder why that is ...*

Needless to say, I performed some hands-on research with Bob Beck's devices and his Protocols. Today, I am pleased to report that the periodic outbreaks that I experienced for twenty years have stopped!!!

Listen, to wait for someone to save you who's paid handsomely not to is insane. After the allopathic plunge, all that the medical establishment has to do to block an important discovery is **NOT TEST IT!** If its not tested, it can't be approved; and if its not approved, *effective or not*, doctors who use it can be put in legal jeopardy. Here's the bottom line: *the Medical Industrial Complex can't keep charging absurd fees for repetitive mediocre treatment, unless they can block your access to effective cures.* **In view of this, please research Energetics with an open mind. I did, and an incurable disease (according to the CDC and medical establishment) which plagued me for decades is no longer a concern in my life!**

Epilogue:

There is a tremendous difference between knowing what you've always been told—and knowing what's true! In fictitious times, to herald the truth is often seen as a revolutionary act, and to champion a paradigm shift—**Abomination**! This all notwithstanding, centuries ago Sir William Drummond was to declare:

> *"He who will not reason is a bigot;*
> *He who cannot is a fool;*
> *And he who dares not is a slave . . ."*

Insomuch as none of these conditions befits a self-actualized person in the 21st century, let me be the first to congratulate and wish you many wonderful, *and rewarding*, discoveries in your investigation of Energetics. IF IT IS CAUSED BY A VIRUS, BACTERIA, OR PARASITE—IT IS TIME TO <u>**STAND UP AND TAKE BACK YOUR LIFE**</u>!!!

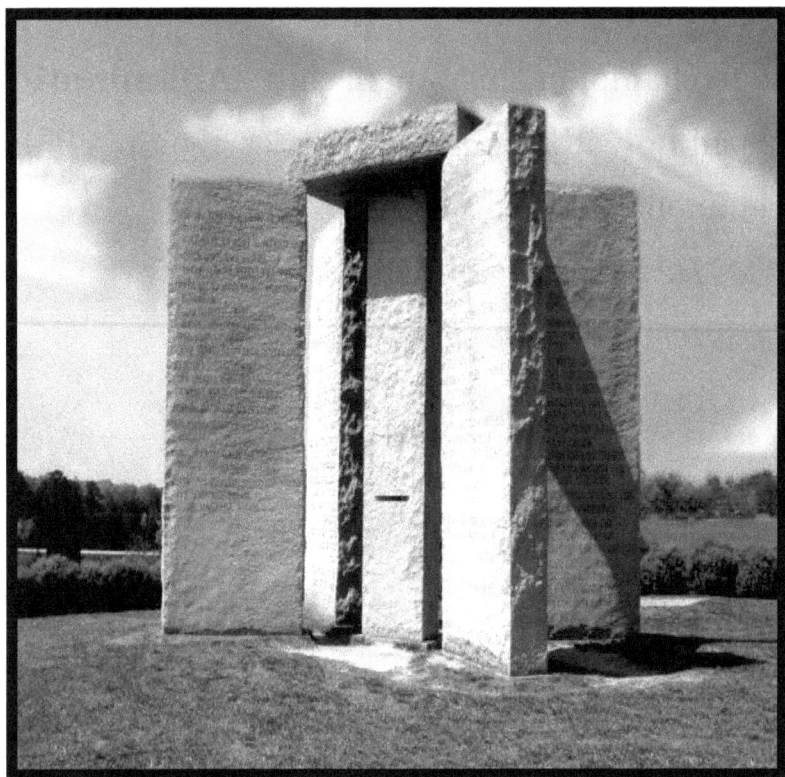

Glossary:

A.M.A.
The AMA's stated mission is to promote the art and science of medicine for the betterment of public health, to advance the interests of physicians and their patients, to promote public health, to lobby for legislation favorable to physicians and patients, and to raise money for medical education. The AMA also publishes a list of Physician Specialty Codes, which are the standard method in the U.S. for identifying physician and practice specialties.

Attenuate
To cause something to become weak.

Bacteria
One-celled organisms, spherical, spiral, or rod-shaped and appearing singly or in chains, comprising the Schizomycota, and commonly involved in fermentation, putrefaction, infectious diseases, or nitrogen fixation.

Benign
A mild disposition or character that does not threaten health or life.

Biological Warfare (Germ Warfare)
The use of pathogens such as viruses, bacteria, other disease-causing biological agents, or the toxins produced by them, as biological weapons (see pages 196 - 197).

Cancer
A malignant tumor of potentially unlimited growth that expands locally by invasion and systemically.

Centers for Disease Control & Prevention (CDC)
United States federal agency under the Department of Health and Human Services, based in Georgia. The stated mission is to protect public health and safety by providing information to enhance health decisions, and it promotes health through partnerships with state health departments and other organizations.

Clone
In biological terms, an asexually reproduced life form.

Disease
An impairment of the normal state of the living animal (or plant body or one of its parts) that interrupts or modifies the performance of the vital functions. Often it is manifested by distinguishing signs and symptoms that are a response to specific infective agents (e.g., worms, bacteria or viruses).

Electricity
A fundamental entity of nature consisting of negative and positive kinds, observable in the attractions and repulsions of bodies electrified by friction and in natural phenomena (as lightning or the aurora borealis) and usually utilized in the form of electric currents.

Electromagnetism
Of, relating to, or produced by electromagnetism. Light, microwaves, x-rays, and TV and radio transmissions are all types of electromagnetic waves.

Energetics
A term which encompasses all fields or disciplines that utilize electromagnetic energy for therapeutic use.

Eugenics
Science of eliminating genetic traits through selective breeding and forced sterilization (see page 198).

Food and Drug Administration (FDA)
An agency of the United States Department of Health and Human Services that is responsible for protecting and promoting public health through the regulation and supervision of food safety, tobacco products, dietary supplements, prescription and over-the-counter pharmaceuticals (medications), vaccines, biopharmaceuticals, blood transfusions, medical devices, electromagnetic radiation emitting devices (ERED), veterinary products, and cosmetics. The FDA also enforces other laws, notably Section 361 of the Public Health Service Act and associated regulations, many of which are not directly related to food or drugs. These include sanitation requirements on interstate travel and control of disease on products ranging from certain household pets to sperm donation for assisted reproduction.

Georgia Guidestones
A monument in Georgia which calls for the death of 90% of the world's population (see page 184).

Germ
A microorganism often associated with a disease.

Illness (Sickness)
An unhealthy condition of body or mind.

Ionization
A physical process of converting an atom or molecule into an ion by adding or removing charged particles such as electrons or other ions.

Malignant
Something that tends to produce death or deterioration; often associated with cancerous tumors.

Microorganisms
An organism that is microscopic or submicroscopic, which means that it is far too small to be seen by the

unaided human eye.

Paradigm

A long and well-established standard. Paradigms maybe correct or incorrect. For instance, despite the fact that the ancient Egyptians and Phoenicians were circumnavigating the earth 2500 years ago, Europeans thought the earth was flat until the 1490s. The arrival of Columbus in the Bahamas was the beginning of their shift from the incorrect flat earth paradigm, to the correct view that the planet is actually round.

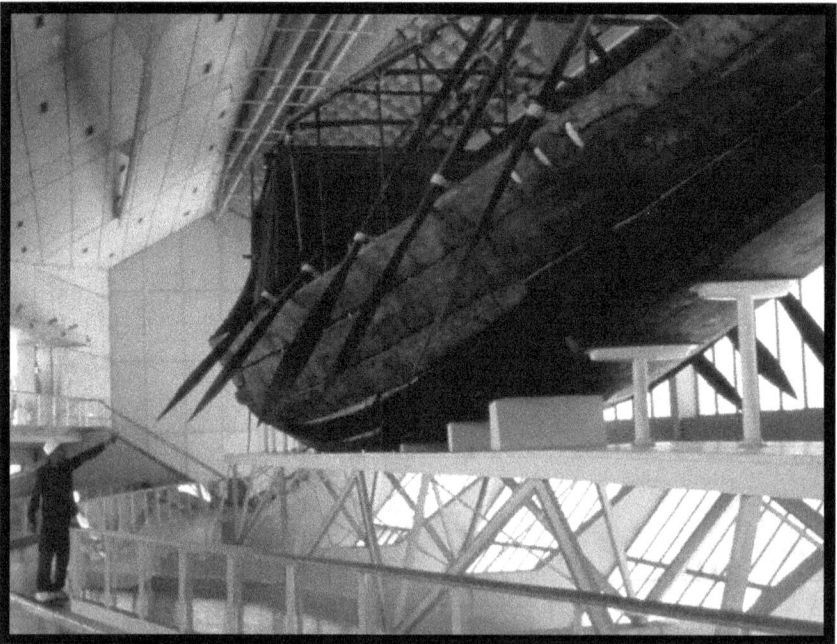

Egyptian Ship c. 2400 BCE – Giza Museum

Parasite

An organism that lives on, or in, an organism of another species (known as the host). The former obtains its life sustaining nourishment from the latter.

Patent

A patent is a set of exclusive rights granted by a national government to an inventor or their assignee for a limited period of time, in exchange for a public disclosure of an invention. The procedure for granting patents, the requirements placed on the patentee, and the extent of the exclusive rights vary widely between countries according to national laws and international agreements. Typically, however, a patent application must include one or more verifiable claims defining the invention which must be new, non-obvious, and useful or industrially applicable. The exclusive right granted to a patentee in most countries is the right to prevent others from making, using, selling, or distributing the patented invention without permission.

Pathogen

Any disease-producing agent is considered to be a

pathogen. The term is commonly associated with viruses, bacterium or other microorganisms.

Pharmaceutical Industrial Complex (also known as Big Pharma and Pharmaceutical Industry)

A 200 billion dollar industry that sells prescription drugs to the public like candy. Bob Beck disclosed the fact that many of the same families involved in selling illegal drugs also control the legal side of the drug business (pharmaceuticals). While personally being in no position to comment about his claim one way or another, I would like to make a few brief observations here insomuch as the scriptures explain, *"A tree is known by its fruit."*

One cannot help but note that some rather interesting parallels exist between the illegal and legal drug cartels:

*First, they both produce drugs that can be highly addictive.

*Second, they both produce drugs that have harmful side-effects (*up to and including death*). For instance, in The Pharmaceutical Industrial Complex Null and Henderson explain that Merck's Vioxx has been responsible for 44,000 deaths and 120,000 injuries.

*And third, they both practice price markup obscenity. While there isn't really any need to discuss the drug profits garnered by illegal drugs—allow me to share these facts about the price markup of the legal pharmaceutical corporations.

Brand Name	Consumer price 100 units	Cost of Generic Active Ingredient 100 units	Percent Markup
Celebrex 100mg	$130.27	$0.60	21,712%
Claritin 10mg	$215.17	$0.71	30,306%
Keflex 250mg	$157.39	$1.88	8,372%
Lipitor 20mg	$272.37	$5.80	4,696%
Norvasc 10mg	$188.29	$0.14	134,493%
Paxil 20mg	$220.27	$7.60	2,898%
Prozac 20mg	$247.47	$0.11	224,973%
Xanax 1mg	$136.79	$0.024	569,958%
Zoloft 50mg	$206.87	$1.75	11,821%

Figures complied by Doug Henderson and Dr. Gary Null

After some reflection on pages 37 – 47 here, it appears that old habits are hard to break. Yet, whereas a century ago the government stopped the monopolists, today it has been usurped to such an extent that its being used to rob and march the citizenry straight back into poverty and serfdom.

Physicist

A scientist who studies matter and energy and interactions between the two, grouped in traditional fields such as acoustics, optics, mechanics, thermodynamics, and electromagnetism, as well as in modern extensions including atomic and nuclear physics, cryogenics, solid state physics, particle physics and plasma physics.

Symptom

Subjective evidence of disease or physical disturbance observed by the patient.

Theoretical

Concerned primarily with theories, speculation and/or hypotheses.

Therapeutic
Of, or relating to, the treatment of disease.

Useless Eaters
The antithesis of God's word that he would *number them like the stars of the heavens and the sands of the seashore*—useless eaters is a pejorative designation for 90% of the world's population by a small group of trillionaires, billionaires and their lackeys. According to documents dating back a hundred years, the aim of this group is to kill or imprison all of the useless eaters on the earth. In 1974, Henry Kissinger said: *"Depopulation should be the highest priority of foreign policy towards the Third World."* Today, this group is calling for the wholesale annihilation of peoples of all races and creeds (see pages 196 - 199). *Don't be deceived, this isn't about resource depletion, the environment, or intellect—it's about greed, insecurity and control.*

Virus
An ultramicroscopic metabolically inert infectious agent that replicates only within the cells of living hosts, mainly bacteria, plants and animals. It has an RNA or DNA core, a protein coat, and, in more complex types, a surrounding envelope.

DEPARTMENT OF DEFENSE APPROPRIATIONS FOR 1970

HEARINGS

BEFORE A

SUBCOMMITTEE OF THE COMMITTEE ON APPROPRIATIONS HOUSE OF REPRESENTATIVES

NINETY-FIRST CONGRESS

FIRST SESSION

SUBCOMMITTEE ON DEPARTMENT OF DEFENSE

GEORGE H. MAHON, Texas, *Chairman*

ROBERT L. F. SIKES, Florida
JAMIE L. WHITTEN, Mississippi
GEORGE W. ANDREWS, Alabama
DANIEL J. FLOOD, Pennsylvania
JOHN M. SLACK, West Virginia
JOSEPH P. ADDABBO, New York
FRANK E. EVANS, Colorado '

GLENARD P. LIPSCOMB, California
WILLIAM E. MINSHALL, Ohio
JOHN J. RHODES, Arizona
GLENN R. DAVIS, Wisconsin

R. L. MICHAELS, RALPH PRESTON, JOHN GARRITY, PETER MURPHY, HOWARD NICHOLS, ROBERT FOSTER, *Staff Assistants*

' Temporarily assigned

H.B. 15090

PART 5

RESEARCH, DEVELOPMENT, TEST, AND EVALUATION

Department of the Army
Statement of Director, Advanced Research Project Agency
Statement of Director, Defense Research and Engineering

U.S. GOVERNMENT PRINTING OFFICE
WASHINGTON : 1969

30-334

Glossary

DEPARTMENT OF DEFENSE APPROPRIATIONS FOR 1970

SYNTHETIC BIOLOGICAL AGENTS

There are two things about the biological agent field I would like to mention. One is the possibility of technological surprise. Molecular biology is a field that is advancing very rapidly and eminent biologists believe that within a period of 5 to 10 years it would be possible to produce a synthetic biological agent, an agent that does not naturally exist and for which no natural immunity could have been acquired.

Mr. SIKES. Are we doing any work in that field?

Dr. MACARTHUR. We are not.

Mr. SIKES. Why not? Lack of money or lack of interest?

Dr. MACARTHUR. Certainly not lack of interest.

Mr. SIKES. Would you provide for our records information on what would be required, what the advantages of such a program would be, the time and the cost involved?

Dr. MACARTHUR. We will be very happy to.

(The information follows:)

The dramatic progress being made in the field of molecular biology led us to investigate the relevance of this field of science to biological warfare. A small group of experts considered this matter and provided the following observations:

1. All biological agents up to the present time are representatives of naturally occurring disease, and are thus known by scientists throughout the world. They are easily available to qualified scientists for research, either for offensive or defensive purposes.

2. Within the next 5 to 10 years, it would probably be possible to make a new infective microorganism which could differ in certain important aspects from any known disease-causing organisms. Most important of these is that it might be refractory to the immunological and therapeutic processes upon which we depend to maintain our relative freedom from infectious disease.

3. A research program to explore the feasibility of this could be completed in approximately 5 years at a total cost of $10 million.

4. It would be very difficult to establish such a program. Molecular biology is a relatively new science. There are not many highly competent scientists in the field, almost all are in university laboratories, and they are generally adequately supported from sources other than DOD. However, it was considered possible to initiate an adequate program through the National Academy of Sciences-National Research Council (NAS-NRC).

The matter was discussed with the NAS-NRC, and tentative plans were made to initiate the program. However, decreasing funds in CB, growing criticism of the CB program, and our reluctance to involve the NAS NRC in such a controversial endeavor have led us to postpone it for the past 2 years.

It is a highly controversial issue and there are many who believe such research should not be undertaken lest it lead to yet another method of massive killing of large populations. On the other hand, without the sure scientific knowledge that such a weapon is possible, and an understanding of the ways it could be done, there is little that can be done to devise defensive measures. Should an enemy develop it there is little doubt that this is an important area of potential military technological inferiority in which there is no adequate research program.

Source: Department of Defense Appropriations for 1970. Hearings Before a Subcommittee of the Committee on Appropriations House of Representatives, Ninety-First Congress, Tuesday, July 1, 1969, Page 129. Washington: U.S. Government Printing Office, 1969.

ENERGETICS

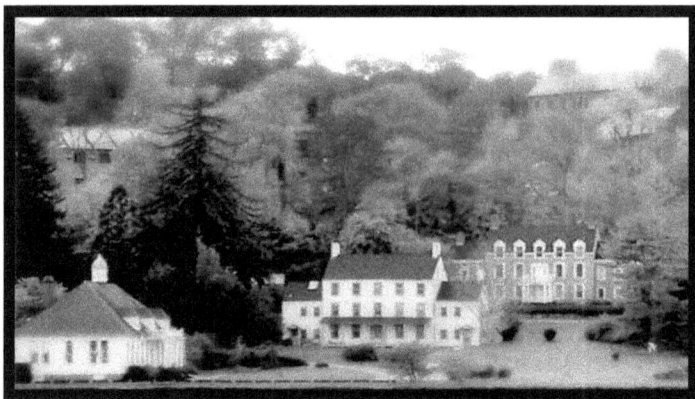

Cold Spring Harbor Laboratory

About the same time that the recommendations of the Flexner Report were being implemented across the country, eugenics research was also being funded by John D. Rockefeller, Mary Harriman and the Carnegie Institution at Cold Spring Harbor Laboratory. Charles Davenport and Harry Laughlin headed the eugenics program. In 1910, the nation's first Eugenics Records Office (ERO) was established on the CSHL estate in New York.

The principal push of the ERO and the CSHL was to make compulsory sterilization the law of the land. By the 1920s, many state legislatures had introduced bills to legalize forced sterilization. The following states passed compulsory sterilization laws: Arizona, California, Connecticut, Delaware, Georgia, Idaho, Iowa, Kansas, Maine, Michigan, Minnesota, Mississippi, Montana, Nebraska, New Hampshire, North Carolina, North Dakota, Oklahoma, Oregon, South Carolina, South Dakota, Utah, Vermont, Virginia, West Virginia, and Wisconsin.

While the most widely stated goal was to use forced sterilization to stop the "feeble minded" or "mentally retarded" from procreating, the motive for the work of many eugenicists was based upon their racial, and xenophobic, agendas. For example, prominent eugenicists were behind the immigration legislation of the 1920s, which limited the numbers of Eastern Europeans, Asians and Italians from entering the United States. The eugenicists also backed segregation and laws against interracial marriage. During the 20th century, the sterilization targets of the eugenicists would include the following: orphans of all races (a-r), the poor, homeless, and disabled (a-r), violent criminals (a-r), prostitutes (a-r), alcoholics (a-r), Africans, Native Americans, Russian and Polish immigrants, and the elderly in Germany.

Although the science of the early eugenicists was eventually discredited, many prominent Americans would extol the virtues of eugenics: The Rockefeller Foundation, Theodore Roosevelt, A. Lawrence Lowell, David Starr Jordon, Lothrop Stoddard, Vernon Kellogg, Alexander Graham Bell, Luther Burbank, Madison Grant, Margaret Sanger, and H.J. Webber to name a few. It must be noted here that one of the celebrated founders of the ERO, Harry H. Laughlin, would eventually be diagnosed with epilepsy; thereby, placing him in the inferior gene stock pool, which made him an ERO compulsory sterilization designee! Needless to say, Laughlin was not so zealous in his support for forced sterilization when it came to himself and his family . . .

It is estimated that about 65,000 people were forced to undergo compulsory sterilization in the United States. Truth be told, the Nazis who were tried for War Crimes at Nuremberg testified that they used the policies of American eugenicists at the CSHL, as the basis for their eugenics program. Of course, the Nazis would go on to kill and/or sterilize millions. Today, Cold Spring Laboratory is the site of America's Human Genome Project.

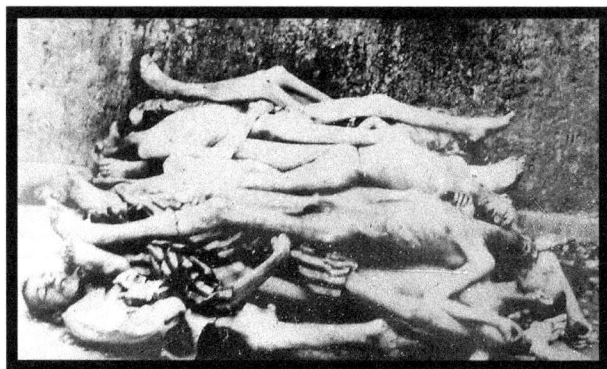

Mass Grave at Buchenwald 16 April 1945

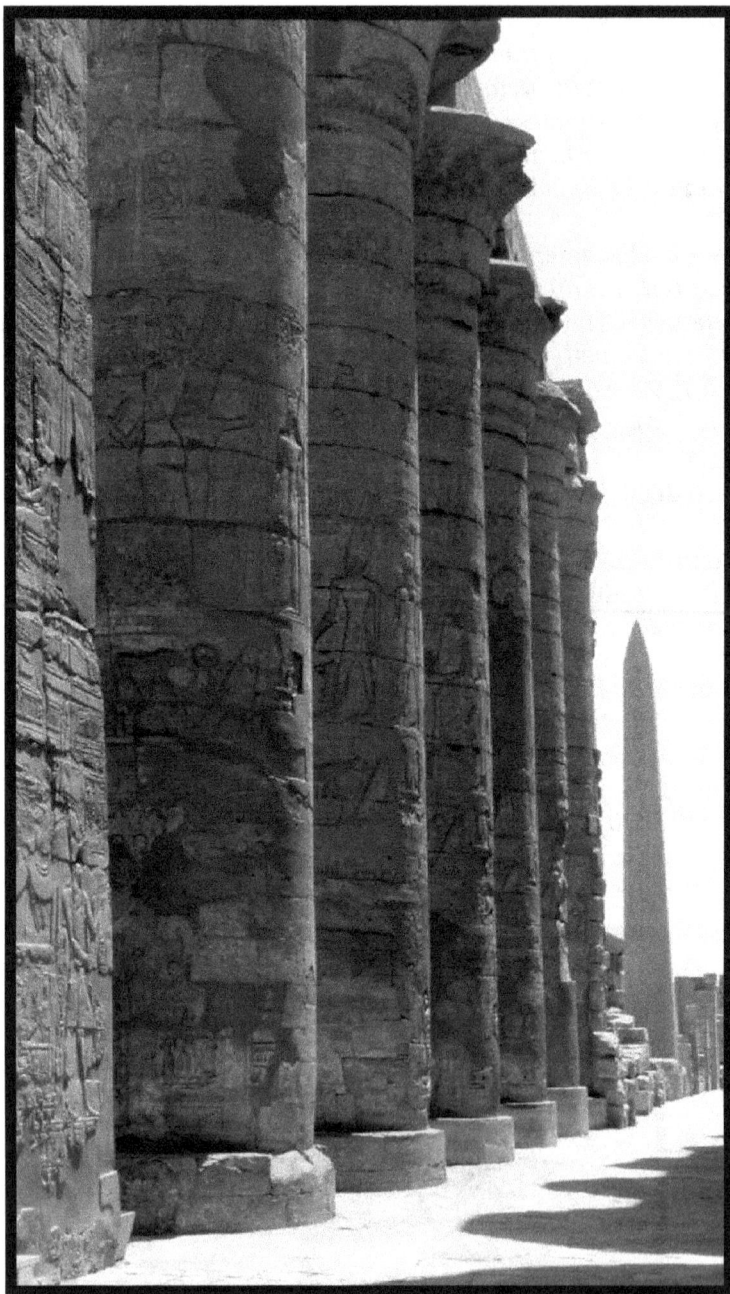

Temple Complex of Amen-Ra in Egypt

Glossary

<u>The Physician's Cardinal Rule</u>

*F*rom time to time, modern medical professionals will loftily refer to the Hippocratic Oath. This usually happens when the need arises to quell some public concern over a medical misstep. With health care industry cost at an all-time high—and no decline in the number of patients who are actually being harmed by doctors and drug companies in sight—one can expect the pill pushers and the corporate media to provide even more allusions to this reassuring oath in the coming years . . .

Yet, when it came to health care in the days of the first physicians, healing was not approached as a profession—but a reverent calling! These men and women were students of life, whose charge was to only engage a vessel of the divine when it was in distress—and through that interaction, return the person back to health (wholeness). ATOP THAT, <u>THE CARDINAL RULE OF AN ANCIENT PHYSICIAN WAS TO **DO NO HARM**</u>*!* Amongst the ancients, this maxim was no public relations tool, it was a time-honored convention that was cherished and enforced: <u>Diodorus explaining that a physician who caused a death by failing to follow protocol could actually be put on trial for his life!</u> While nobody is calling for this today, one can't help but be struck by the impunity given to medical professionals and drug companies who injure, <u>and even kill</u>, hundreds of thousands of people annually (see pages 30 – 32).

Today, we are a long way from the spirit of the world's first physicians. For instance, amongst the Egyptians (who were the actual inspiration for the Hippocratic Oath) money was the furthest thing from a doctor's mind. Indeed, many physicians were paid laborers' wages. Such a wage is not that surprising once stopping to reflect upon the fact that, philosophically speaking, for an Egyptian—<u>the idea of becoming wealthy from the suffering of others would be seen as the height of moral and physical insensitivity!</u> Accordingly, we learn that the kingdom's treasury regulated and paid the cost of medical care for all Egyptians. This structure allayed patient doubt as to the motivation for the treatments that doctors prescribed. Finally, on the preceding page we have the ancient Egyptian Temple Complex of Amen-Ra at Thebes. This renowned complex is the largest ancient religious site in the world! I thought it fitting to close with it here forsomuch as De Lubicz explains that this complex was not just a group of religious buildings—but a timeless spiritual monument to the anatomy of man as well: organs and vital centers of the body actually being commemorated in many temple structures! Nothing accentuates the contrast between the mental constructs of a healer and a mechanic more . . . (See note page 53)

201

Photo Credits:

Unless otherwise stated, all images courtesy of The Hall of Records - KornerStone Books ©

Page 3 – Public Domain Artwork by Daniel Mytens: <u>William Harvey</u>

Page 9 – <u>Imhotep</u> *appears courtesy* Hu Totya *A.S.A. 3.0* Wikipedia

Page 11 – Public Domain Artwork by Philippe de Champaigne: <u>Cardinal-Duc de Richelieu</u>

Page 13 - Public Domain Artwork by Sculteti: <u>Armamentium Chirugiae</u>

Page 17 – Public Domain Artwork by Gilbert Stuart: <u>George Washington</u>

Page 20 – Public Domain Artwork by Hans von Gersdorff ?: <u>Amputation</u>

Page 22 – National Archives & Records Admin: <u>No. 36 Amputation at Gettysburg 1863</u>

Page 28 – Public Domain Artwork: <u>Christian Friedrich Samuel Hahnemann</u>

Page 34 – Public Domain Photo: <u>Obama Health Care Speech before the Joint Session of the 111th Congress</u> - USGov

Page 38 – Public Domain Rockefeller Archive Ctr: <u>John D. Rockefeller</u>

Page 39 – National Archives & Records Admin: <u>Ludlow Strikers Funeral</u>

Page 50 – Public Domain Artwork by Brumidi: <u>The Apotheosis of Washington</u>

Page 103 – <u>HIV</u> *appears courtesy* C. Goldsmith – USGov-HH-CDC

Page 104 – <u>Plasmodium falciparum</u> *appears courtesy* USGov-HH-CDC

Photo Credits: {cont}

Photo Credits: {cont}

Page 150 – <u>Tomb of Lionus</u> appears *courtesy* Soprintendenza Archeologica Etr. Merid. Plazza Di Giulia

Page 152 – <u>Robert Koch</u> *appears courtesy* USGov-NIH

Page 155 – <u>Crystal glass</u> *appears courtesy* Acoustics, Audio and Video Group, University of Salford - www.acoustics.salford.ac.uk

Page 161 – Public Domain Artwork by Aubin Millin: <u>Ophiuchus & the Serpent Bearer</u> - Museo Pio Clements Rome

Page 162 – <u>Temple of Dendera</u> *appears courtesy* Mr. Lasse Jensen CC-BY-2.5. Wikipedia

Page 178 – <u>Herpesviridae</u> *appears courtesy* USGov-HHS-CDC

Page 184 – Public Domain Photo: <u>Georgia Guidestones</u> *appears courtesy* Picoterawatt

Page 193 – <u>Big Pharma Chart</u> - *data compiled by* Null, G., & Henderson, D., The Pharmaceutical Industrial Complex: A Deadly Fairy Tale

Page 196 - 197 – <u>House Bill 15090</u> *appears courtesy* USGov - & Horowitz, L., & Puleo, J., Healing Codes for the Biological Apocalypse

Page 198 – <u>Cold Spring Harbor Laboratory</u> *appears courtesy* AdmOxalate CC-BY-3.0 Wikipedia

Page 199 – <u>Buchenwald 16 April 1945</u> *appears courtesy* Jule Rouard - Luc Viatour GNU Free Documentation License 1.2 Wikipedia

Bibliography:

Adams, G., Doctors in Blue Schuman 1952

Armstrong, J., The Water of Life Vermilion 1971

Arora, N., Eugenics Record Office Shunya
http://www.shunya.net/Text/Blog/eugenics.htm 2010

Bailey, D., & Wright, E., Practical Fiber Optics Elsevier
2003

Bailey, R., William Harvey: Father of Cardio-vascular
Medicine
http://biology.about.com/library/organs/blcircsystem2.htm
2010

Bain, V., & Ma, M., Acute Viral Hepatitis Gastroresource
www.gastroresource.com 2010

Barber, J., Ancient Healing Codes Revealed in Bible
http://www.tetrahedron.org/articles/healing_codes/Healin
g_Codes_Press_Release.html 2010

Bechtel, S., & Stains, L., Sex: A Man's Guide St. Martin's
1996

Beck, B., Bob Beck Lecture: Take Back Your Power (PDF)
1997

Becker, R., & Seldon, G., The Body Electric Morrow 1985

Beckingham. R., ABC of diseases of liver, pancreas, and biliary system: Acute hepatitis BMJ Vol. 322, No. 7279 2001 pp. 151 - 153

Berlitz, C., Atlantis: The Eighth Continent Putnam & Sons 1984

Berlitz, C., Mysteries From Forgotten Worlds Doubleday 1972

Berlitz, C., The Bermuda Triangle Doubleday 1974

Bishop, M., The Horizon Book of the Middle Ages American Heritage & Bonaza Books 1968

Black, E., War Against the Weak Dialog Press 2007

Blayney, K., The Caduceus vs. the Staff of Asclepius http://www.drblayney.com/Asclepius.html 2010

Bowder, D., Who's Who in the Greek World Phaidon 1982

Brennan, H., The Secret history of Ancient Egypt Piatkus 2000

Brock, T., Robert Koch: A Life in Medicine and Bacteriology AMS 1999

Brugsch-Bey, H., & Seymour, H., A History of Egypt Under the Pharaohs Murray 1879

Bruinius, H., Better For All the World: The Secret History of Forced Sterilization and America's Quest for Racial Purity A. Knopf 2006

Bibliography

Bucaille, M., Mummies of the Pharaohs St. Martin's Press 1990

Budge, E.A., The Dwellers on the Nile Dover 1977

Bunson, M., A Dictionary of Ancient Egypt Oxford Univ. 1995

Burn, A., & Selincourt, A., Herodotus the Histories Penguin 1972

Butzer, C., (Ed.)., Ancient Egypt: Discovering Its Splendors National Geographic Soc. 1978

Calladine, C., & Drew, H., Understanding DNA: The Molecule & How IT Works Academic Press 1966

Camp, J., The Healer's Art: The Doctor through History Taplinger 1977

Carlyon, R., Guide to the Gods Heinmann 1981

Carper, J., Food Your Miracle Medicine Harper-Collins 1993

Carter, J., Racketeering in Medicine: The Suppression of Alternatives Hampton Roads 1993

Cartwright, F., Disease and History Crowell 1972

Castiglioni, A., History of Medicine (2d ed.) Knopf 1947

Clark, R., The Sacred Tradition in Ancient Egypt: The Esoteric Wisdom Revealed Llewellyn 2000

ENERGETICS

Clayman, C., The Human Body: An Illustrated Guide to its Structure, Functions, and Disorders Dorling Kindersley 1995

Daily, G., & Ehrlich, P., DEVELOPMENT, GLOBAL CHANGE, AND EPIDEMIOLOGICAL ENVIRONMENT Ctr. For Conservation Biology Stanford Univ. 1995

Dampier-Whetham, W., A History Of Science: And its relations with Philosophy & Religion Macmillan 1931, Cambridge Univ. 1948

Daniel, G., Nubia Under the Pharaohs Westview Press 1976

David, R., The Egyptian Kingdoms Bedrick Books 1990

Davis, A., Women, Race and Class Vintage 1981

De Lubicz, R., Sacred Science: The King of Pharaonic Theocracy Inner Traditions International 1961

De Lubicz, R., The Temple in Man Inner Traditions 1949

Dharmananda, S., ELECTRO-ACUPUNCTURE Institute for Traditional Medicine www.itmoline.org 2010

Dodson, A., Monarchs of the Nile Amer. Univ. 2000

Donnelly, I., & Sykes, E., Atlantis: The Antediluvian World Gramercy 1949

Eckerson, H., Immigration and National Origins Annals of the American Academy of Political and Social Science Vol. 367 1966 pp. 4-14, p.6

Estes, J., The Medical Skills of Ancient Egypt Science History Pub. 1989

Bibliography

Fagg, C., Ancient Greece Warrick Press 1978

Finch, C., Ancient African Medical Practices (Audio) 1992

Fosar, G., & Bludorf, F., Vernetzte Intelligenz Omega 2001

Garratt, A., Medical Electricity Lippincott 1866

Geyman, J., Health Care in America: Can Our Ailing System Be Healed? Butterworth-Heinemann 2002

Ghalioungui, P., Magic and Medical Science in Ancient Egypt Barnes & Noble 1963

Giller, R., Natural Prescriptions: Dr. Giller's Natural Treatments & Vitamin Therapies For Over 100 Common Ailments Random House 1994

Goellnitz, J., Civil War Surgery & Amputation http://ehistory.osu.edu/uscw/features/medicine/cwsurgeon /amputations.cfm 2010

Goldman, J., Holy Harmony (CD) Goldman & Sound Healers Publishing 2002

Hall, M., The Secret Teachings of All Ages The Philosophical Research Soc. 1977

Hallowell, M., Herbal Healing Avery 1994

Heifetz, M., & Tirion, W., A Walk through the Southern Sky Cambridge Univ. 2000

Henderson, D., & Null, G., The Pharmaceutical Industrial Complex: A Deadly Fairy Tale Global Research, October 21, 2009 Progressive Radio Network

ENERGETICS

Henry, W., & Gray, M., Freedom's Gate (DVD) www.williamhenry.net 2010

Heymsfield, S., Lohman, T., Wang, Z., Going, S., Human Body Composition Human Kinetics 2005

Himmelmann, L., From barber to surgeon- the process of professionalization Sven Med Tidskr. Vol. 11, No. 1 2007 pp. 69 - 87

Hobson, C., The World of the Pharaohs Thames & Hudson 1982

Horowitz, L., DNA: Pirates of the Sacred Spiral (DVD) New Science Ideas 2005

Horowitz, L., Emerging Viruses and Vaccinations DVD NSI 2006

Horowitz, L., The American Red Double-cross http://www.tetrahedron.org/articles/apocalypse/red_doubl e_cross.html 2010

Horowitz, L., & Puleo, J., Healing Codes for the Biological Apocalypse Tetrahedron 2006

Janssen, R. & Janssen, J., Growing Up in Ancient Egypt Rubicon Press 1990

Johnson, R., Atomic Structure Twenty-First Century 2007

Kühl, S., The Nazi Connection: Eugenics, American Racism, and German National Socialism Oxford University Press 2002

Bibliography

Lakhovsky, G., Curing Cancer with Ultra Radio Frequencies Radio News 1925

Lakhovsky, G., & Clement, M., Secret of Life: Cosmic Rays and Radiations of Living Beings William Heinemann 1939, Mokelumme Hill 1970

Laughlin, H., Eugenical sterilization in the United States Psychopathic Laboratory of the Municipal Court of Chicago 1922

Levin, M., Current and potential applications of bioelectromagnetics in medicine ISSEEM Journal Vol. 4, No. 1, 1993 pp. 77 - 87

Lynes, B., Cancer Solutions: Rife, Energy Medicine and Medical Politics Elsmere Press 2000

Lynes, B., The Cancer Cure That Worked: Discovery and Suppression of the Cancer Cure That Worked! Marcus Books 2005

Malek, J., & Forman, W., In the Shadow of the Pyramids Univ. of Oklahoma

Maspero, G., History of Egypt The Grolier's Soc. 1901

Maver, W., Electricity, its History and Progress, The Encyclopedia Americana; a library of Universal knowledge Vol. X Encyclopedia Americana Corp. 1918

McGrew, R., Encyclopedia of Medical History McGraw Hill 1985

Mendelsohn, R., Confessions of a Medical heretic Contemporary Books 1979

Michon, G., Scientific Symbols and Icons: The staff of Aesculapius
http://www.numericana.com/answer/symbol.htm 2010

Mindell, E., & Hopkins, V., Prescription Alternatives McGraw-Hill 2009

Morris, S., Life's Solution: Inevitable Humans in a Lonely Universe Cambridge Univ. 2003

Morton, D., 10 Excruciating Medical Treatments from the Middle Ages   http://www.oddee.com/item_96620.aspx 2010

Moscati, S., The Face of the Ancient Orient Dover 2001

Muller, M., Mythology of All Races Vol. XII Cooper Square 1964

Mullins, E., Murder by injection: the story of the medical conspiracy against America National Council for Medical Research 1992

Murphy, E., Diodorus on Egypt McFarland 1985

Nardo, D., Atoms Kidhaven Press 2002

Null, G., Prescription for Disaster DVD Null & Assoc. 2005

Null, G., & Dean, C., & Feldman, M., & Rasio, D., & Smith, D., Death By Medicine LE Magazine http://www.lef.org/magazine/mag2006/aug2006_report_death_01.htm 2010

Oates, J., Babylon Thames & Hudson 1979

Bibliography

Osler, W., The Evolution of Modern Medicine (e-book) GUTENBERG 1913

Paul, D., Controlling Human Heredity, 1865 to the Present Humanities Press 1995

Peltier, L., Fractures: A History and Iconography of their Treatment Norman 1990

Proctor, R., Racial Hygiene: Medicine Under the Nazis Harvard University Press 1988

Rogers, J.A., Sex and Race Rogers Pub. 1967

Rondberg, T., Under the Influence of Modern Medicine Chiropractic Journal 1998

Ropes, L., Aristotle Black Inc. 1943

Sadek, A., History of Medicine - Some Aspects of Medicine in Pharaonic Egypt AAMS January 2001

Saunders, J., The Transitions From Ancient Egyptian to Greek Medicine Univ. of Kansas 1963

Schultz, S., William Harvey and the Circulation of the Blood: The Birth of a Scientific Revolution and Modern Physiology News in Physiological Science Vol. 17, No. 5, Oct. 2002 pp. 175-180

Sedgewick, W., Tyler, H., & Bigelow, R., A Short History of Science Macmillan 1939

Seigworth, G., Bloodletting Over the Centuries NEW YORK STATE JOURNAL OF MEDICINE Dec. 1980, pp. 2022-2028

Smith, W., Dictionary of Greek and Roman Biography and Mythology Murray 1880

Sonntag, L., Sensational Sex Hamlyn 2000

Starfield, B., Is US Health Really the Best in the World? JAMA Vol. 284, No. 4, July 26, 2000 pp. 483-485.

Stetter, C., The Secret Medicine of the Pharaohs Quintessence Pub. 1993

Sturridge, E., Dental Electro-therapeutics Lea & Febiger 1914

Sullivan, D., A Short History of Eugenics (PDF) http://soulfulbioethics.blogspot.com 2010

Taton, R., History of Science Basic Books 1965

Tesla, N., & Childress, D., The Fantastic Inventions of Nikola Tesla Adventures Unlimited 1993

Thornwald, J., Science and Secrets of Early Medicine Harcourt, Brace & World 1963

Tompkins, P., The Magic of Obelisks Harper & Row 1981

Vadakan, V., A Physician Looks At The Death of George Washington Early America Review: Archiving Early America http://www.earlyamerica.com/review/2005_winter_spring/washingtons_death.htm 2010

Van Sertima, I., Blacks in Science: Ancient and Modern Transactions 1983

Van Sertima, I., They Came Before Columbus R. House 1977

Bibliography

Warren, L., Did Ancient Cultures know about Electricity? Plim Report http://www.plim.org/scienceapr97.html 2010

Williams, N., Death of Dolly marks cloning milestone Current Biology Vol. 13, No. 6 Mar. 2003 pp. 209 - 210

Wilson, J., Culture of Ancient Egypt Phoenix Books 1951

Worthy, R.L. About Black Hair KornerStone 2006

Worthy. R.L. The Racialization of Slavery KornerStone 2009

Worthy, R.L., YHSVH KornerStone 2008

Zahoor, A., Hospitals and Medical Schools in the Dark and Middle Ages http://cyberistan.org/islamic/sibai10.html 2010

Zinn, H., A People's History of the United States HarperCollins 2006

_____., Ancient Lives (VHS) Spry-Leverton & WTTW 1984, 1988

_____., Arthur Clarke's Mysterious World: Ancient Discoveries (VHS) Discovery Chan. 9/21/87

_____., Bioelectromagnetic Medicine Taylor 2007

_____., Bobby Lee Show: Murder by Injection Interview E. Mullins Lee Video prod. 1993

_____., Cholera: a Deadly Infection Bukisa http://www.bukisa.com/articles/368702_cholera-a-deadly-infection 2010

ENERGETICS

_____., CIA World Factbook 18 December 2003 to 18 December 2008

_____., Coil For Electromagnets Twenty First Century Books http://www.tfcbooks.com/patents/coil.htm 2010

_____., Electronics 101: Fundamentals of Electricity http://www.electronicstheory.com/html/e101-1.htm 2010

_____., Elephantine Museum - Artifact Collection

_____., Encyclopedia of Medical History McGraw Hill 1985

_____., Encyclopedia of Religion Macmillan 1987

_____., Essential Atlas of Physiology Barron's 2005

_____., Fativa: Ancient Healing Codes Revealed in Bible Are Published by Tetrahedron Press http://Factiva.com 1999

_____., Global Sciences Congress: THE BOB BECK INTERVIEW http://www.health-science-spirit.com/beckinterview.html 2010

_____., History of Barbering Barberpole.com 2010

_____., NationMaster www.NationMaster.com 2010

_____., New World Encyclopedia http://www.newworldencyclopedia.org/entry/Caduceus 2010

_____., Sicko Michael Moore & Megan O'Hara (DVD) 2007

Bibliography

_____., The Beck Protocol Sharing Health (DVD) 2001

_____., The Granada Forum: Suppressed Medical Discovery (DVD) Transformation Technologies 1997

_____., The Old Kingdom and First Intermediate Period (PDF) Cleveland Museum of Art (?)

_____., The Strecker Memorandum (VHS) The Strecker Group 1988

_____., The World Book Encyclopedia The World Book Encyclopedia 1959

_____., The World's Strangest UFO Stories O'Sullivan & Evans 2006

_____., Twenty First Century Books: Coil For Electromagnets 2010

_____., Universal Standard Encyclopedia W. Funk 1955

_____., Wikipedia: Eugenics http://en.wikipedia.org/wiki/Eugenics 2010

_____., World Development Indicators 2002 (CD-ROM) Washington, DC World Bank 2002

_____., World Health Organization: Health Statistics 2010 http://www.who.int/entity/whosis/whostat/EN_WHS10_Full.pdf 2010

_____., Xenophilia: The Rife Microscope Cancer Cure Story www.xenophilia.com/zb0012.htm 2011

Index:

A

Acupuncture   156
AIDS   25
56–58, 102–103, 114, 176,
180
Amen-Ra   7
200-201
American Medical
Association (AMA)   44
45, 51, 114, 187
Amputation   14
19-22, 24
Antibiotics   29
Antibodies   159
Apotheosis   50
51
Aristotle   23
Asclepius   161
163
Aurelius, M.   151

B

Baghdad Battery   149
163
Barber pole   15-16
21
Barbers   14
16, 19-23
Beck, B.   ix
47-48, 54–100, 115, 147,
156, 158, 176, 180–181, 194
Biological Warfare
(Germ Warfare)   186
Blake, W.   155
Blood
Electrification   57
58, 102, 112, 149, 158, 180-
181
Bloodletting   12–18
21, 24
Brumidi, C.   51
Buchenwald   199
Butler, S.   167

C

Caduceus   51-53
Cancer   vii
47-48, 58, 130–131, 154,
156, 188
Capitol   50-51
Cardinal Rule   201
Carter, J.   50
Catholic Church   11-14
CDC   35
179, 181, 188
Chakra   164
Cholera   173
Chronic Fatigue   58
Civil War   21-22
Cloning   142–143
189
CNN   58
114
Coffman, M.   174
Coitus   170
Cold Spring
Harbor Laboratory   41-42
198-199
Colitis   29
Confucius   59

Congress   47
51
Corporate Media   29
31-32, 174
Crohn's Disease   33
Culling   174

D

Daily, G.   172-173
Defibrillator   158
Diarrhea   105
DNA   133
135-141
Dolly
the Sheep   142-143
Drummond, W.   183

E

Egyptians   2
4–9, 23, 138, 147–151,
162–165, 169, 192, 200 -
201

Ehrlich, P. 172-173
Etruscans 150
Eugenics 43
188, 190, 198-199
Eustulin, D. 174

150
Greeks 2
7, 9, 163-164, 201
Gymnarchus
Niloticus 150

F

FDA 58
112, 190
Feces 172–173
175
Finsen, N. 154
Flexner, A. 42-45
Flexner Report 41-45
198
Fox 114

G

Galen 12
Georgia Guidestones 184
191
Gout 148

H

Hahnemann, C.S. 27-29
Harvey, W. 3–5
10, 12, 24
Health Care
Budget 48
201
Health Care
Rankings 49
Hepatitis vii
58, 174
Herpes vii
58, 176, 178-181
Hippocrates 5
201
HIV vii
56-58, 102- 103, 176, 179-180
Holistic 37

Homeopathic   29
37
Horowitz, L.   41-42
133 – 135, 137-138, 141,
174
Human Genome
Project   41
199

I

Icke, D.   174
Illingworth, C.   113–114
125-127
Imhotep   9
52, 163-164
Immortal Blood   59
Ionic Medicine   126
Ionization   118-127

J

Johnson, M.   154
167

Jones, A.   174

K

Kaali, S.   25
56–57, 115, 156
Kissinger, H.   195
Koch, R.   152
Kundalini   164

L

Laibow, R.   174
Lakhovsky, G.   129–132
135, 141, 143–144, 153, 179
Laminitis   122
Laughlin, H.   198-199
Levin, M.   127
Lionus   150
Lorenzen, L.   137-138
Ludlow Massacre   39
Lupus   58
Lyman, W.   25
56–57, 156

Lyme Disease 58

M

Malapterurus
Electricus 148
Malaria 104
Measles 107
Mendelsohn, R. 48
52-53
Meningitis vii
110
Mercury 51
Mesopotamia 2
23, 150
Mi (528 Hz) 137
Monteith, S. 174
Mortal Oscillatory
Rate (M.O.R.) 154
Mullins, E. 39
46-48

N

Navy, U.S. 55

Nazis 199
Nemes, Dr. 167
Nobel Peace Prize 58–59
154
Null, G. 30
32

O

Obama, B. 34
Ophiuchus 160-164

P

Paul 55
Pharmaceutical
Industry 46
129, 194-195, 201
Pliny 150
Pneumonia 29

Q

R

Rameses II 146
149
Richlieu, Cardinal 11
Rife, R. 153–155
160, 167, 179
Rockefeller, J. 37-47
198-199
Rockefeller, W. 40
Rome 7
150-151

S

Sawbones 21-22
Schwolsky, P. 115
156
Scotland 151
September 11th 31
Sinyukhin, A. 133
141
Solomon 165

Soul 143-144
Starfield, B. 30
Strecker
Memorandum 179
Syphilis 111

T

Temple of Hathor
at Dendera 162-163
TENS Machine 150
Tesla, N. 127
139 – 141, 147, 153, 179
Tetanus 109
Thebes 201
Torpedo
Marmorata 148
Tuberculosis 106
Tucker, J. 174

U

Ultra Sound 56
Ultraviolet Light 156

U.S. Patent Office   102
115, 132, 156-157
Useless Eaters   174
197

V

Vaccinations   10
31, 112-114

W

Wands of Horus   149
151
Washington, G.   16-18
24, 48, 50-51
Whopping Cough   108
Wild, J.   156
Winfrey, O.   58
Wright, J.   174

Y

Z

X

ENERGETICS
Discount Order Form

Of course, you can call any of your local bookstores and ask them to order a copy of Energetics for $39.95 plus tax. You should be able to pick your copy up in 48-hours. However, if you would like to have a copy (or copies) delivered to your doorstep and save money—just go to **www.korner-store.com** to order online *via* PayPal for the discount sale price of $34.95! Or, photocopy this page and use it as an order form. Just fill in the information and mail the discount sale price of $34.95 per book to the address below (money orders please). You should receive your order one week after processing. For orders of 5 books or more - contact us via email to learn about our volume discounts!

Name:_____

Address:_____

City, State & Zip:_____

Number of Books:_____   Amount Enclosed:_____
{No sales tax outside of WA. State}

KornerStone Books
6947 Coal Creek Pkwy.
Suite 206
Newcastle, WA. 98059
sales@korner-store.com

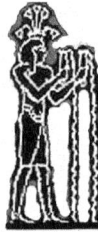

Insomuch as Man means Mind–
To refuse to engage the latter, is to fail to become the former . . .